PAIN MANAGEMENT

Advances in Diagnosis & Treatment

2011 Report

A Special Report published by the editors of
Arthritis Advisor
in conjunction with
Cleveland Clinic

Pain Management: Advances in Diagnosis & Treatment

Consulting Editor: Nagy Mekhail, MD, PhD, Chairman, Department of Pain Management, Cleveland Clinic

Author: Jim Brown, PhD

Group Directors, Belvoir Media Group: Diane Muhlfeld, Jay Roland

Creative Director, Belvoir Media Group: Judi Crouse

Associate Editor, Belvoir Media Group: Kristine Lang

Production: Mary Francis McGavic

Publisher, Belvoir Media Group: Timothy H. Cole

ISBN: 1-879620-80-4

To order additional copies of this report or for customer service questions, please call 877-300-0253, go to www.arthritis-advisor.com/products, or write to Health Special Reports, 800 Connecticut Avenue, Norwalk, CT 06854-1631.

This publication is intended to provide readers with accurate and timely medical news and information. It is not intended to give personal medical advice, which should be obtained directly from a physician. We regret that we cannot respond to individual inquiries about personal health matters.

Pain Management
Advances in Diagnosis & Treatment

There have been many promising advances in pain management this year, but four areas that have received special attention are the genetic connection to pain, the benefits of exercise in reducing pain, improving coping mechanisms, and the better understanding of how healthcare providers can successfully manage and treat chronic pain.

Multi-disciplinary and highly-specialized approaches to chronic pain are gaining more popularity and much more success. This is when a specialized clinic is established that addresses special chronic pain problems by multiple specialists at the same time to produce an individualized comprehensive treatment program. For example, cancer pain patients are to be evaluated by an oncologist, a palliative care specialist, and a pain management physician. Chronic abdominal or pelvic pain patients should be evaluated by a gastrointestinal or gynecology specialist, in addition to the pain management specialist. Also, chronic pediatric pain should be evaluated by a pediatrician, psychologist, and pain physician who specializes in pediatric pain.

Other multidisciplinary approaches include techniques such as acupuncture, meditation, and relaxation and seem to be effective for some patients. It also appears that the presence of a specific type of gene may make some people more susceptible to chronic pain, which could lead to different strategies in treating them. Recognizing these connections will help pain management professionals develop patient-specific therapies that hasten their return to a more normal life.

Pain Management 2011 has been updated and some segments have been added or completely rewritten to include breaking developments, but the information is still organized in a way that makes it easy for you to read, understand, and use.

Chapter 1 goes beyond an explanation of the pain process and provides practical information about pain and depression, stress, genetics, gender, aging, and falls. Chapter 2 describes and updates 17 conditions that could predispose a person to chronic pain, including a new section on chronic pelvic pain syndrome. Chapter 3 discusses more than two dozen traditional pain management approaches, and Chapter 4 provides the latest information on 15 complementary and alternative strategies. Chapter 5 covers methods of helping to control chronic pain through exercise, diet, and weight control. It illustrates strength and stretching exercises, tells you how to determine your target heart rate, and walks you through a 12-week exercise program.

Help is more available than ever for people suffering from chronic pain, and Chapter 6 tells you how to find a pain management specialist, how to prepare for your first office visit, and what to expect when you get there. At the back of the book you'll find a list of pain management resources and contact information and an expanded glossary of 68 terms.

Cleveland Clinic Department of Pain Management Chairman Nagy Mekhail, MD, PhD, and his colleagues believe this newest edition of *Pain Management* will be a valuable resource for patients and caregivers.

■ ■ ■

HIGHLIGHTS

■ Depression leads to "over-remembering" of pain. (Page 11, Box 1-2)

■ Word association may add to pain sensation. (Page 12, Box 1-4)

■ Presence of gene may cause some people to be more sensitive to pain. (Page 13, Box 1-5)

■ "Accidentally reprogrammed" genes may cause chronic pain. (Page 13, Box 1-6)

■ Chronic pain contributes to falls among older adults. (Page 15, Box 1-7)

■ Aerobic exercise eases symptoms of fibromyalgia. (Page 23, Box 2-4)

■ Migraine headaches linked to heart disease. (Page 24, Box 2-5)

■ Naproxen, acetaminophen may provide migraine relief. (Page 25, Box 2-6)

■ Aspirin may relieve migraine pain in 25-50 percent of patients. (Page 25, Box 2-7)

■ Cognitive behavioral therapy may relieve chronic back pain. (Page 35, Box 3-1)

■ Duloxetine reduces lower back pain for certain patients. (Page 38, Box 3-3)

■ Not all NSAID meds equal in risk of internal bleeding. (Page 39, Box 3-5)

■ Opioid pain medications increase risk of fractures. (Page 40, Box 3-6)

■ TENS not recommended for long-term low-back pain. (Page 42, Box 3-7)

■ Acupuncture deactivates area of brain associated with pain. (Page 53, Box 4-1)

■ Evidence weak for acupuncture treatment of fibromyalgia. (Page 54, Box 4-2)

■ Electroacupuncture for 30 minutes affects pain perception. (Page 55, Box 4-4)

■ Chiropractic treatment using multiple approaches relieves back pain for some. (Page 56, Box 4-5)

■ Magnetic stimulation offers treatment option for migraine patients. (Page 60, Box 4-6)

■ Meditation may bring pain relief. (Page 61, Box 4-7)

■ Slow breathing techniques may reduce moderate pain. (Page 63, Box 4-8)

■ Activity improves function, reduces pain of fibromyalgia. (Page 64, Box 5-1)

■ Lower back-specific exercises relieve chronic back pain. (Page 65, Box 5-2)

■ Lack of exercise, obesity increase osteoarthritis risk in women. (Page 69, Box 5-13)

■ Obesity elevates risk of fibromyalgia pain. (Page 69, Box 5-14)

TABLE OF CONTENTS

Pain Management:
Advances in Diagnosis & Treatment
2011 Report

INTRODUCTION

The numbers are staggering. More than 75 million Americans—one in every six adults—report problems with persistent, long-term, chronic pain. For older adults, the numbers are even more troubling. By the age of 65, half of us will have some degree of chronic pain, often caused by ailments such as arthritis, back and neck pain, shingles, or headaches. Chronic pain occurs in as many as 90 percent of cancer patients. The economic impact of chronic pain is an upwardly mobile target, but estimates begin at $60 billion per year.

In too many cases, we don't know what causes our pain. To make matters worse, most of us wait an average of a year or longer before seeking help. Chronic pain is the country's most under-reported and under-treated condition.

But pain does not have to be quietly endured, and it doesn't have to go untreated. Nagy Mekhail, MD, PhD, Chairman of the Department of Pain Management at Cleveland Clinic, says that chronic pain is a disease—not a symptom—that can be treated and managed. "We have diagnostic and therapeutic options available so that you do not have to accept chronic pain as a way of life."

Dr. Mekhail and his colleagues at Cleveland Clinic, as well as others at pain management centers of excellence around the country, work with medical specialists and healthcare professionals to find the source of your pain and develop a plan specific to your circumstances.

The most important member of your pain management team is you. Instead of being a passive recipient of treatment, you must become part of the team that solves the problem. Patients who wait

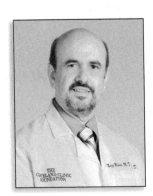

Nagy Mekhail, MD, PhD, Chairman, Department of Pain Management, Cleveland Clinic

at home, hoping for a medical miracle, are not as likely to improve as those who make decisions regarding the foods they eat, the amount of exercise they get, the kinds of medications they take or avoid, and even the company they keep.

Today, we understand that chronic pain is common, costly, and complex. It is not part of the natural aging process, and it is individual in nature. The question is, "What will you do about it?" We hope that you will start by using the information in *Pain Management 2011* to help yourself, the people you care for, and those who might care for you.

1 PRACTICAL APPLICATIONS

The day-to-day effects of chronic pain vary from person to person and are associated with physical or emotional stress, even when the cause remains the same. What is debilitating pain to one person may be a minor problem for another.

Acute pain is usually a warning signal for an underlying disease, inflammation, or injury and comes on suddenly as a sharp pain or ache. The most important feature of acute pain is its cause-and-effect relationship to the injury or inflammation. The pain is felt as long as the source of the pain is still there. In contrast, chronic pain is a disease by itself. There is no definite cause-and-effect relationship to injury or inflammation. Early, effective treatment of acute pain may prevent a conversion of the condition to a chronic pain syndrome.

Chronic pain has staying power. If a condition takes two or three weeks to improve and the person still has pain three months later, the pain is considered chronic. In contrast to acute pain, the cause-and-effect relationship between the injury and the pain sensation is lost. Long after the immediate danger has passed, the warning signal continues to sound.

Patients and their doctors now understand that chronic pain has both physical and psychological components. The psychological makeup of the patient can have an effect on the way pain is perceived, as well as on the success or failure of the treatment. And even if psychological factors don't play a significant role in the early stages, chronic pain eventually takes a tremendous toll on the patient. Anxiety, anger, insomnia, limited physical ability, and depression are real possibilities, making it even more important to include an experienced pain psychologist as part of the chronic pain management team.

We know that chronic pain can linger indefinitely, is a separate disease process that primarily involves the nervous system, does not serve a biological function, and can result in anxiety, fear, and depression.

A series of events

Pain involves a series of events that take place along the pathway of the nervous system. The first action involves the peripheral nerves, a vast network of fibers that encompasses the whole body. These fibers have millions of nerve endings called nociceptors that can sense uncomfortable sensations such as pressure, burns, and cuts, while other types of nociceptors detect inflammation caused by injuries, diseases, or infection. When these sensitive nerve endings detect something that is harmful, they send electrical impulses through the spinal cord by way of chemical messengers called neurotransmitters.

Undamaged nerve fibers, rather than those damaged by injury or disease, may be the cause of pain. Chronic pain makes the neurons (nerve cells) at the level of the spinal cord super-sensitive. Excessive pain response could be the result of this neuron hypersensitivity. Spontaneous pain is caused by the firing of damage-detecting neurons. The reason for the reaction appears to be inflammation within the nerves or tissues. As a result, researchers are now trying to develop new medications that target undamaged nerve fibers. These drugs could eventually affect conditions such as back pain, neuropathy secondary to diabetes, post herpetic neuralgia, or interstitial cystitis.

The speed at which signals are sent to the brain varies with the type of pain. Signals move toward a section of the spinal cord called the dorsal horn, which is essentially a gatekeeper for the central nervous system (see Box 1-1).

All of the messages try to get through the gate, but the special nerve cells of the dorsal horn have a way of filtering the pain messages. For severe, emergency, or life-threatening pain, the gate opens wide, and the message goes through immediately. Lesser pain signals may be blocked or delayed.

Chronic pain is not a slower-moving version of acute pain. Because pain signals are repeated over long periods of time, the nerve cells in the spinal cord change and become hypersensitive to the signals. The type of pain that lingers after the original injury is called neuropathic pain and affects one in 12 people over the age of 55. The damaged nerves, not the original injury, are causing the pain. What should have been a temporary condition becomes a permanent or "chronic" change in the nervous system. Nerve pain is hard to diagnose because the pain results from abnormally functioning nerves inside the body, not from an injury outside the body. Some of the words and phrases that are used to describe neuropathic pain are 'pins and needles,' 'stabbing or burning,' 'numbness,' 'electric-shock-like,' 'walking on glass,' and 'tingling.'

Three developments in the past three years have affected the treatment of neuropathic pain. First, researchers at Washington University in St. Louis identified a gene that

BOX 1-1: PAIN SIGNALS

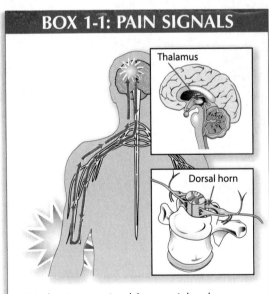

Thalamus

Dorsal horn

Pain begins as a signal from peripheral nerves, which is sent to the dorsal horn. From there it is filtered and relayed to the thalamus and other areas of the brain, which forward signals to the areas responsible for physical sensation.

plays a role in triggering neuropathic pain. The study had an immediate effect on neuropathic pain associated with cancer chemotherapy, as well as the treatment of diabetes, kidney disease, and viral infections. By identifying the gene, doctors may soon be able to prescribe a drug that will offset the blocking mechanism before neuropathic pain develops.

Then the American Academy of Neurology published guidelines for detecting the exact cause of neuropathic pain. The guidelines suggest that patients with nerve pain should discuss screening tests with their doctors that would determine levels of blood glucose, vitamin B12, and serum protein. Genetic testing should be conducted for neuropathic problems that run in families, as well as tests to measure the function of small nerve cells that control sweating, heart rate, and blood pressure. The combined results of all these tests could determine the exact source of neuropathy.

Thirdly, researchers in Boston developed the StEP test that enables physicians to distinguish between neuropathic pain and non-neuropathic pain. The series of tests may soon allow physicians to design treatment strategies instead of speculating about which treatment is most likely to relieve pain.

If and when the bad news—that is, the pain signal—gets to the thalamus in the brain, it does some additional sorting and switching before sending the message to specialized areas—the physical sensation region, the region that handles emotions, and the part that does the serious thinking. Multiple regions of the brain are involved in determining the location of pain.

Chronic pain involves a combination of sensing, feeling, thinking, and past experience. In acute pain states, the brain immediately starts sending its own messages back down through the nervous system to begin the healing process, whether to limit the flow of blood in response to a cut, increase the rate of circulation to get oxygen or nutrients to a stressed area, or release chemicals that suppress pain. With chronic pain, those reverse messages do not always work their way back down the nervous system. In the case of fibromyalgia, for example, the nervous system is not as efficient in sending signals from the brain to block pain.

Pain and the brain

The brain-body connection can determine how much, how often, and for how long something hurts. Chronic pain may even disrupt important mental functions such as attention and memory. Think of pain as your body's all-in-one burglar and fire alarm system. Sometimes it signals danger and is vital for survival. At other times pain is more of a false alarm than a five-alarm emergency. Then there are occasions when the alarm keeps sounding even when the danger has long passed.

You can do several things to block some of the pain messages that would normally get to the brain. The first is to educate yourself regarding your situation. Understanding the diagnosis, the condition, and why you have the pain establishes a foundation for doing something about it.

You can also train your brain in distraction techniques, such as breathing exercises, meditation, yoga, and tai chi. By relieving stress, these activities also relieve pain. Physical distractions include the use of heat, cold applications, changing body positions, and exercise, even if only for five or six minutes at a time. Walking to enhance mobility, stretching to improve range of motion, and using weights to increase strength are all consistent with the mind-body approach to reducing pain.

Probably the most powerful and challenging pain-reducing tool at your disposal is your ability to avoid automatically thinking the worst about the situation that is causing your pain. People who anticipate the worst have lower levels of pain tolerance than those who think more positively. Pain management experts recommend that you acknowledge pain as a challenge, and then do something concrete to manage it effectively. Patients who accept the existence of chronic pain are more likely to have increased emotional, social, and physical function.

The way to make pain worse is to do nothing but sit around and think about it. Pain loves that kind of attention and will stay as long as you will let it. Using brain imaging, scientists have found that positive thinking actually can shape the experience of pain. Decreasing the expectation of pain can reduce both the pain-related brain activity and the perception of pain intensity. Positive thinking could be an important adjunct to managing chronic pain.

You have the ability to change your attitude toward pain from negative to positive. Most people can feel better if they are satisfied that the evaluation of their pain has been thorough, and their doctor has confirmed that they don't have a serious medical problem. Moving toward a positive attitude is especially important to avoid secondary problems such as depression. Chronic pain can affect some people so severely that they need assistance from someone with a fresh outlook—someone who can teach them the tricks of the pain-management trade.

People react to pain in different ways. Not only is there a difference from person to person, but pain awareness also can vary within the same individual. Some patients can function very well even when they perceive their pain at a very high level. Others are unable to function although the actual sensation of pain is very low.

Pain and depression

As many as 40 percent of people with chronic pain experience clinical depression, which can lead to loss of sleep, weight gain or loss, digestive problems, sadness, guilt, and hopelessness. Depression is a separate medical condition, and it can be treated successfully. Physicians frequently overlook depression and anxiety when patients show symptoms of physically disabling conditions such as chronic lower back pain.

Now we know that depression appears to interfere with a person's recollection of pain. A study conducted at the University of Iowa and reported in the October 15, 2009, edition of *Psychosomatic Medicine* found that, in 109 female subjects, those who had higher scores on a test to measure depression were more likely to exaggerate the frequency of their symptoms (see Box 1-2).

Chronic pain may actually cause a change in the way the brain is wired, which may explain why these people have high rates of depression. The area of the brain that is associated with emotion (including depression) appears to be in a constant state of activity, rather than slowing down when other parts of the brain are active.

Medications used to treat depression might not be effective in managing chronic pain. Because pain and depression are often observed in the same patient, doctors are inclined to group the two conditions in terms of treatment. There has been an impression that if you treat the depression, it will make the pain better. But a study of fibromyalgia patients found that a person's level of depression had little influence on the intensity of his or her pain. The authors concluded that pain and depression should be treated separately.

Chronic pain tends to feel more intense when people are sad than when they are happy, even when the pain level is the same. In older adults, pain appears to contribute to greater stress and more serious symptoms of depression. Pain patients who are satisfied with the amount of social support they are getting feel less depressed and are more likely to take action to cope with their pain. Some of the signs of depression include irritability; loss of interest in activities; increased or decreased appetite; chronic fatigue; difficulty thinking clearly, concentrating, or making decisions; and thoughts of death or suicide.

NEW FINDING

Box 1-4: Word association may add to pain sensation

At the University of Jena in Germany, biologists and psychologists investigated how healthy subjects processed words associated with experiencing pain. Using functional magnetic resonance tomography, they found that words alone are capable of activating the brain's pain matrix, and the results suggest that verbal stimuli have a more important meaning than previously thought. It is possible that even speaking often with their physicians or therapists might intensify the pain experience, but other studies will be needed to clarify that possibility. (PAIN, March 30, 2010)

Pain and stress

Stress is normal. Some stressors are positive and some are negative, but either way, your body and mind are built to handle them. The key is to recognize stress and do something about it in a way that does not result in or worsen chronic pain. Pain caused by osteoarthritis, for example, is processed in the same part of the brain that controls stress. This suggests that treatment should address the psychological, as well as the physical aspects of pain.

Individuals with high levels of anxiety due to chronic pain experience more emotional distress and disability, and that anxiety is a strong predictor of depression.

If you are not sure of the exact cause of your stress, it may be helpful for you to know the warning signs. Once you can identify the signs, you can learn how your body responds to stress, and you can take steps to reduce it.

Many of the traditional and alternative therapies discussed in this report address stress reduction. But there are practical ways to deal with stress that do not require counseling or professional care (see Box 1-3).

Pain and anticipation

The anticipation of pain actually can enhance pain, and for some people, anticipating pain is as bad as experiencing it. There is a place in the brain that is activated when you anticipate pain. When that area is activated, more pain information is allowed into the system, and your ability to regulate that pain is deactivated. Remember that gate in the spinal column? It's the dorsal horn and the nerve cells that filter pain messages. Whether all of those messages really make it to their destination depends on the person. A "why me?" attitude throws the gate wide open. A positive state of mind, combined with education about the nature of your pain and the use of distraction techniques, helps to close the gate.

Even words may affect the anticipation of pain. Psychologists in Germany used magnetic resonance tomography to measure patients' brain reactions when they heard words to describe pain. They observed "clear activation" of the pain centers in the brain when pain-associated words were used. The results appeared in the March 30, 2010, edition of the journal *PAIN* (see Box 1-4).

Pain and genetics

Some people may be more sensitive to pain than others. A study in the online March 8, 2010, edition of the *Proceedings of the National Academy of Sciences* reported the presence of a particular gene—SCN9A—in patients who report higher levels of pain than the normal population (see Box 1-5). The study advances the understanding of pain and may lead to more effective treatment.

The journal *Genome Research* reported in its May 6, 2010, issue that chronic pain may be caused by accidental reprogramming of more than 2,000 genes in the peripheral nervous system. The new finding could result in the development of drugs that treat pain by altering the activity of specific genes (see Box 1-6).

Pain and gender

The differences between men and women are now thought to extend to the way they feel, react to, and even describe pain. Gender affects the way different parts of the brain respond in reaction to pain. Brain scans used to measure the reaction of men and women who were subjected to the same pain stimulus have found greater activity in the emotion-based centers of female brains, as opposed to more activity in analytical regions of male brains.

Women appear to be at an elevated risk for developing several chronic pain conditions. Individuals with irritable bowel syndrome may not be able to turn off a part of the brain that controls pain. Women are also more sensitive to pain than men, and their anxiety may be partly responsible for the difference in their pain response. Women appear to respond better than men to chronic pain treatment.

Researchers disagree on some points, but they all agree that pain is a complex process involving physical, psychological, and social factors. One researcher says that women have thinner skin and a higher density of nerve fibers than men, both of which could explain greater sensitivity to pain. Another physical attribute in women—estrogen, a natural painkiller—influences their response to pain in many ways. Fluctuations in hormonal levels could contribute to pain tolerance at various times during the menstrual cycle, during pregnancy, and immediately after childbirth, as well as during and after menopause. In other words, a woman's ability to withstand pain is always changing, and may explain why they can deal with the seemingly unbearable pain of childbirth.

Men and women are even different in the way they report pain. Although women may feel pain more intensely, as some experiments have shown, they may be better at describing their pain to researchers and doctors. An explanation as to why men and women describe pain differently is that our culture puts pressure on men to deny pain, whereas women are expected to be more open about it.

Research tells us that, compared to men, women experience more pain, use more pain-relieving medications, recover from pain more quickly, discuss pain more often, seek help sooner, and use a wider variety of coping strategies. Because of these differences, a treatment that is effective for one gender may not be as effective for the other.

Pain and aging

Chronic pain appears to increase with age. It is the leading complaint of older Americans and its consequences are more profound than in younger adults. Here is the supporting evidence:

- Approximately 25 percent of the Western population is over the age of 70, and that proportion will continue to increase.
- At least 50 percent of elderly adults, not including those living in nursing homes, suffer from significant pain.
- Up to 80 percent of residents in nursing homes have under-treated pain that affects their quality of life.
- More than 25 percent of nursing-home residents with daily cancer pain receive no pain-relieving drugs.
- Increasing age, frailty, and cognitive impairment all increase the risk of under-treatment for pain and illness.

The bodies of older adults process pain medicines differently. Kidneys become smaller with age, blood flow is diminished, and they become a less-effective filtration system to remove a drug. The liver also gets smaller and receives less flow of blood than that of a younger body. This makes it harder for the liver to break down medicines. Oral drugs might be poorly absorbed because of changes in stomach acid levels.

Simply administering drugs to elderly people also can become a challenge. Decreased saliva might interfere with swallowing, and injections might be more difficult because of decreased muscle mass.

There are numerous misconceptions about pain and aging. For example, some say that pain is a normal part of the aging process. Not true. Pain in older adults is not normal and is usually associated with a medical problem.

Another myth is that as people get older, their ability to sense and perceive pain decreases. The truth is that a person's ability to feel pain remains the same throughout life.

It is also untrue that if a person does not complain of pain, he or she must not be in pain. For many reasons, older adults do not always tell others about their pain. Often, they simply don't want to bother anyone. One of the most difficult misconceptions to overcome is that exercising is dangerous if you have pain. Instead, exercise actually helps to prevent muscle wasting and, in some cases, it can reduce pain by making the muscles stronger.

Social interaction is one of the most important components of managing chronic pain in older adults. Those who are involved in social activities and have social connections tend to have a more positive attitude and greater success in managing their pain.

Older patients might be reluctant to report pain, in part because they fear additional tests and excessive costs, or because they are concerned that pain may indicate the progression of a disease. Many wish to be seen as 'good patients' or do not want to take time out of an office visit to report pain.

Report pain to your doctor! Treatments are available. One of the mainstays in pain management for seniors has been the nonsteroidal anti-inflammatory drugs (NSAIDs); however, because these medications can have side effects including stomach irritation and gastrointestinal bleeding, the American Geriatrics Society has established guidelines for pain management that encourage alternatives to aspirin, ibuprofen, and other NSAIDs. The guidelines recommend acetaminophen (Tylenol or Datril, for example) as the first-line treatment for mild-to-moderate pain for seniors. Consult your physician regarding how much Tylenol and other over-the-counter medications you can take per day.

Severe pain may require opium-based drugs such as codeine or morphine. However, older patients are sometimes limited to non-opioid drugs or weak doses, even when their pain is severe. This happens in spite of the fact that, when properly administered, opioid analgesics appear to be safe and appropriate for severe pain in aging adults.

Pain and falls

New research shows that chronic pain often leads to falls, which are the leading cause of death among older Americans. A study published in the November 24, 2009, issue of the *Journal of the American Medical Association* found that 40 percent of the participants said they had chronic pain in more than one joint, while 24 percent reported pain only in one joint (see Box 1-7). More than half of the respondents reported falling at least once during an 18-month follow-up. The study shows that chronic pain that is not addressed can have serious consequences. ■

NEW FINDING

Box 1-7: Chronic pain contributes to falls among older adults

Chronic pain leads to functional decline, muscle weakness, and falls among older Americans, according to a study conducted at Beth Israel Deaconess Medical Center in Boston. Researchers examined the records of 749 people over the age of 70 to determine if a relationship existed between pain and falls. Forty percent of the subjects reported suffering from chronic pain, and 55 percent had fallen at least once during an 18-month period. Having pain during one month increased the risk of a second fall the following month by 77 percent. Researchers now have a better understanding of the connection between pain and falls, and they have new evidence to encourage falls prevention programs among patients and their physicians. *(Journal of the American Medical Association,* November 24, 2009)

2 IDENTIFYING POSSIBLE CAUSES

Long-term pain can be caused by a combination of physical and psychological factors, which can make a diagnosis difficult. Chronic pain is not imagined. It is real and its consequences are profound for the patient, the patient's family, friends, and caregivers.

Many diseases and conditions can result in chronic pain. Your pain management physician can make a diagnosis and develop a treatment plan by becoming familiar with your full medical history, identifying your symptoms, thoroughly examining the affected areas of your body, obtaining X-rays, imaging scans, or other investigations. Your pain specialist might require doing diagnostic nerve blocks to pin down the exact source and mechanism of your chronic pain.

This chapter discusses chronic pain-producing ailments, their causes, symptoms, and risk factors. Treatment options are discussed more extensively in Chapters 3 and 4. The conditions are arranged alphabetically with the areas of the body most likely to be affected (see Box 2-1).

Arthritis (Osteoarthritis)
Areas most likely affected: fingers, thumbs, neck, lower back, knees, and hips

Osteoarthritis (OA) is the most common of more than 100 types of arthritis, affecting an estimated 27 million people. Osteoarthritis causes joint cartilage to break down or wear out. The bones under the cartilage rub against each other, causing pain, swelling, and limitation of motion. The body tries to heal the damage done by osteoarthritis, but it doesn't do a very good job. Often the result is new bone growth (bone spurs) that looks lumpy and may cause tenderness and pain.

OA, also called degenerative joint disease, is a particular problem for older adults. More than half of people over age 65 show evidence of osteoarthritis in at least one joint. Nearly half of all Americans will develop knee osteoarthritis during their lifetime, and that the highest risk is among those who are obese.

Before age 45, the condition is more common in men; after age 45, it is more prevalent in women. By the age of 75, more than 80 percent of Americans either have symptoms or X-ray evidence of OA. Although unsure of what causes the disease, scientists suspect a combination of factors, including being overweight, aging, joint injury, and stress due to work-related or sports activities. People who have had a previous joint injury, who are obese, or who have a family history of OA are most likely to develop the condition.

The symptoms of OA depend on which part of the body is affected. Because the knees are the body's primary weight-bearing joints, they are often susceptible to OA. Stiffness, swelling, and pain can make it difficult to walk, climb, and get in and out of chairs and bathtubs. If not treated, osteoarthritis of the knees can lead to disability. Osteoarthritis in the hips causes pain, stiffness, and severe disability. Activities such as moving and bending are limited, making even a simple act like getting dressed a challenge. Those who have the condition can feel pain in their hips, groin, buttocks, or knees. Spinal osteoarthritis causes stiffness and pain in the neck or in the lower back, as well as weakness or numbness in the arms and legs.

Osteoarthritis does not always cause the affected area to become painful. In fact, only a third of people whose X-rays show evidence of arthritis report pain or other symptoms.

BOX 2-1: CAUSES OF CHRONIC PAIN AND AREAS AFFECTED

CONDITION	MOST LIKELY AFFECTED AREAS
Arthritis (Osteoarthritis)	Fingers, thumbs, neck, lower back, knees, hips
Arthritis (Rheumatoid)	Wrists, hands, feet, ankles
Cancer	Any part of the body
Chronic pelvic pain syndrome	Pelvic region below navel, between hips
Complex regional pain syndrome	Arm, leg, hand, foot
Facet joint pain	Back, neck, shoulders
Fibromyalgia	Neck, shoulders, back, hips, legs
Headaches	Head, neck, sinuses
Herniated disc	Lower back, neck
Irritable bowel syndrome	Abdomen, stomach
Osteoporosis	Spine, hips, wrists
Sciatica	Lower back, buttocks, legs
Shingles	Waist, sides, face
Spinal stenosis	Back
TMD/TMJ	Jaw, head, ear, face
Trigeminal neuralgia	Head, face, jaw
Trigger points	Upper back, neck

The following are warning signs of OA from the National Institutes of Health:

- Constant or intermittent aching pain in a joint
- Stiffness after getting out of bed or sitting for a long time
- Swelling
- Tenderness
- A crunching feeling or the sound of bone rubbing against bone

Treatment for OA includes exercise, weight control, rest, medications, alternative therapies, joint injections, and surgery.

Arthritis (Rheumatoid arthritis)
Areas most likely affected: wrist, hands, feet, ankles

Rheumatoid arthritis (RA) is the most debilitating type of arthritis. About two million people in the United States have rheumatoid arthritis, but some studies show that the number is diminishing. RA affects all races and ethnic groups, often beginning between the ages of 20 and 50, but it can develop in children and young adults as well. Two to three times as many women get RA as men.

RA is an inflammatory disease and is also thought to cause the body's immune system to attack the lining of the joints. Scientists are still not sure why this happens, but it could be associated with genetic factors, environmental conditions, or hormonal changes in women.

RA progresses through three stages: 1) swelling in the lining of the joints, 2) rapid division and growth of cells that cause the lining to thicken, and 3) inflamed cells that release enzymes. The enzymes digest bone and cartilage, causing joints to lose their shape and alignment, and affecting movement (see Box 2-2).

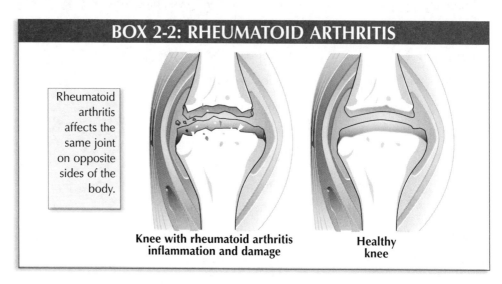

BOX 2-2: RHEUMATOID ARTHRITIS

Rheumatoid arthritis affects the same joint on opposite sides of the body.

Knee with rheumatoid arthritis inflammation and damage

Healthy knee

Symptoms of RA include:

- Tender, warm, swollen joints
- Same joint affected on both sides of the body (both wrists, for example)
- Joint inflammation in the wrist and finger joints closest to the hand
- Fatigue
- Fever
- Sense of not feeling well
- Pain or stiffness for more than 30 minutes in the morning or after a long rest
- Symptoms that last for years

Early treatment for RA can limit joint damage and the resulting loss of movement. Treatment focuses on minimizing damage, controlling pain, and reducing inflammation through a combination of drugs, usually including methotrexate. A modified-release form of prednisone appears to be more effective at reducing morning joint stiffness than the standard version of the steroid. Injections, physical therapy, exercise, and surgery are other treatment options. Changes in symptoms must be monitored closely (at least every two to four months) and treatment changed accordingly.

It may be possible to identify women at high risk of RA by a blood test. Elevated levels of two proteins in the blood appear to be reliable biomarkers of RA long before symptoms appear.

Cancer
Areas most likely affected: any part of the body

Cells normally grow and divide when and where in the body they are needed. The distinguishing characteristic of cancer is uncontrolled cell growth. Malignant tumors crowd out healthy cells, interfere with body functions, and steal nutrients away from the tissues that need them. Cancer spreads through a process called metastasis and can form new tumors in other parts of the body. Below are the four most common forms of cancer and the areas of the body where they originate.

Type of cancer	Points of origin
Carcinoma	Skin, lungs, breasts, pancreas, other organs
Sarcoma	Bone, muscle, cartilage
Lymphoma	Lymphatic system
Leukemia	Blood

Pain associated with cancer can be caused by the disease, the treatment (including chemotherapy or radiation therapy), or both. Between 30 and 50 percent of people with cancer experience pain caused by the treatment, and

70-90 percent of those with advanced stage cancer report pain from the disease itself. Tumors may put pressure on organs, bones, or nerves, and they can obstruct the bowels or the flow of blood. Chemotherapy, radiation, and surgery used to treat cancer all produce side effects, which can include discomfort.

The important point to remember is that cancer pain, regardless of the cause, can and should be managed. More than 90 percent of cancer patients with chronic pain are able to successfully control their pain. Both chronic pain and episodes of acute pain ('breakthrough pain') can be eased with medications. Ten to fifteen percent of cancer patients may require aggressive interventions/surgery to control their pain.

Chronic pelvic pain syndrome
Areas most likely affected:
pelvic region below navel, between hips

Chronic pelvic pain (sometimes referred to as chronic pelvic pain syndrome) has historically been associated with women, but it can also occur in men. The common denominators are pain in the front part pelvic region that can be dull, sharp, steady, or intermittent. Causes among women could include, among other things, long-term infection and endometriosis. In men and women, chronic pelvic pain could be caused by irritable bowel syndrome, interstitial cystitis, or muscle spasms, all possibly compounded by psychological factors such as depression or stress. In men, the symptoms are often related to the intestines or urinary tract that mimic those of prostatitis, such urinary frequency, urgency, difficulty in starting, erratic flow, and pelvic floor pain.

Another common characteristic of chronic pelvic pain syndrome among both men and women is the difficulty in getting an accurate and timely diagnosis. It often involves a process of elimination that might take months or years, and should include a thorough medical history, physical exam, and laboratory tests, as well as imaging when needed. During or even after that period of time, treatment might involve antibiotics (if infection has been detected), prescription and over-the-counter pain medications, relaxation exercises, physical therapy, and in rare cases, surgery. In cases where no specific cause can be found, the goal of treatment may be to manage your pain.

Complex regional pain syndrome
Areas most likely affected: arms, legs, hands, feet

Although it doesn't matter to the patient in practical terms, there are two types of complex regional pain syndrome (CRPS). Type 1 results from irritation of the peripheral and central nervous system without evidence of nerve damage. The condition might be precipitated by trauma, surgery, and even, in rare cases, injections. Type 2 CRPS is the same as Type 1 with evidence of peripheral nerve damage.

Relentless, intense pain that is out of proportion to the severity of an injury might be CRPS, which used to be called reflex sympathetic dystrophy (RSD). While not the most common cause of chronic pain, it is one of the most classic and least understood forms, affecting women at twice the rate of men. CRPS most often affects a single arm, leg, hand, or foot. It gets worse over time, and the pain might spread to the entire arm or leg. The possible symptoms include:

- Intense, burning pain
- Skin sensitivity
- Swelling
- Color changes in the affected area
- Increased skin temperature in early cases; decreased temperature in advanced cases
- Sweating
- Atrophy and loss of function of the limb (in late stages)

There is no cure for CRPS. The goal of treatment is to rehabilitate the limb to avoid loss of function, while trying to control the symptoms. Analgesics, antidepressants, corticosteroids, opioids, nerve blocks, spinal or peripheral nerve stimulation, and drug infusion pumps are a few of the drug-related treatment options. All of those measures give temporary relief, at best. Spinal cord stimulation is a relatively new technology that provides substantial long-lasting relief to a good percentage of CRPS patients for whom other therapies fail to relieve symptoms. Physical therapy and nerve blocks are other options. Nothing will produce a long-lasting solution in every patient, although CRPS recedes into spontaneous remission in some people. The best outcome is achieved if this condition is treated as early as possible in the course of the disease. Researchers are studying ways to intervene more aggressively following a traumatic injury to prevent it from developing into CRPS.

Facet joint pain
Areas most likely affected: back, neck, shoulders

Facets are small, smooth, bony parts of the vertebrae in the back that extend outward to form joints. These joints only move a few

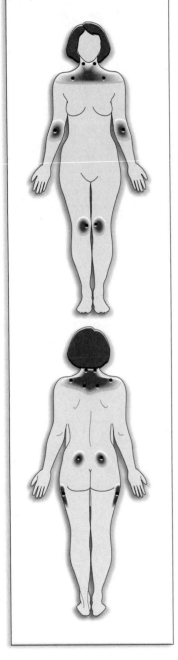
millimeters to allow us to extend our back or neck and rotate from side to side, but when that movement is restricted, it can lead to pain and limited range of motion. The underlying cause of facet joint pain is not always known. Trauma, degeneration, osteoarthritis, and previous spine surgery are all possibilities.

The site of inflammation can be very tender to pressure because the capsule of the facet joints contains nerves. Severe pain occurs when the surrounding muscles become involved. If the dysfunctional facets are between the shoulder blades, the pain can radiate up to the shoulders and neck. The condition is more likely to occur in the upper part of the spinal column than in the lower back, but it can develop in either area. Treatment options include rest, mobilization of the joint, anti-inflammatory drugs, muscle relaxants, exercises, and injections, which affect the joint itself and/or block the ablation of the nerves that supply the joint.

You may not be able to prevent facet joint pain, but stretching your shoulders and upper body can help relieve it. Shoulder shrugs are one type of strengthening lift that should be on your list of stretches. (Shrugs are illustrated in Chapter 5.)

Fibromyalgia

Areas most likely affected: neck, shoulders, back, hips, legs

Fibromyalgia is a common and chronic condition that is characterized by widespread muscle pain and multiple tender points on the neck, shoulders, back, hips, and upper and lower extremities when pressure is applied to them (see Box 2-3).

Characteristically, these tender points vary in severity from one day to another. One day they can be more severe in the shoulders, another day more severe in the lower back and legs. Most of the 3 to 6 million people who have fibromyalgia are women. Most are diagnosed during middle age, but symptoms can develop earlier. People with rheumatoid arthritis, lupus, and spinal arthritis are more likely to develop fibromyalgia than people who don't have these conditions. Fibromyalgia also has been associated with physically or emotionally stressful events such as car accidents, repetitive use injuries, and illnesses. Although the exact cause is still a mystery, there is evidence that the brains of people with fibromyalgia are more sensitive to pain.

Some people consider fibromyalgia to be an arthritis-related condition, but it is not a true form of the disease. It can cause pain and fatigue, but it does not inflame or damage joints, muscles, or other tissues.

In addition to pain and fatigue, other symptoms of fibromyalgia include:

- Headaches
- Irritable bowel syndrome
- Memory problems
- Morning stiffness
- Numbness or tingling of the extremities
- Painful menstrual periods
- Restless legs syndrome
- Sleep disturbances
- Temperature sensitivity

People with fibromyalgia typically see many doctors before getting a diagnosis. Once the condition has been identified, a team approach (doctor, physical therapist, and other specialists) seems to work best. Drugs commonly recommended for fibromyalgia include analgesics, nonsteroidal anti-inflammatory drugs (NSAIDs), antidepressants, and benzodiazepines (such as Valium). Patients treated with the drug pregabalin (Lyrica) appear to have as much as a 50 percent reduction in pain. Milnacipran (Savella) has been approved after clinical trials showed a possible 30 percent reduction in pain, and researchers at Stanford reported that a low dose, inexpensive drug called naltrexone was effective in treating chronic pain in a small sample of women. Antidepressants may be able to ease some of the symptoms of the condition.

Fibromyalgia can last a lifetime, but it's not fatal, and the condition improves over time in many people. To minimize the impact of the condition, get enough sleep, exercise regularly, make changes in your work environment (fewer hours, less demanding responsibilities, and a more comfortable workstation), and eat a well-balanced diet. Walking, strength training, and stretching may reduce symptoms of fibromyalgia. A study published in the May 10, 2010, issue of *Arthritis Research & Therapy* found that light-to-moderate intensity land or water-based exercise significantly reduced pain and fatigue, while it elevated mood and improved fitness (see Box 2-4).

Headaches

Areas most likely affected: head, neck, sinuses

There are many types of headaches, and each has its own causes, symptoms, and treatments. The most important element in correctly diagnosing headache is listening to the patient's history of the pain. Where does it

---

NEW FINDING

Box 2-4: Aerobic exercise eases symptoms of fibromyalgia

Researchers studied the records of more than 2,400 patients in 28 separate trials to determine the effect of aerobic exercise on the symptoms of fibromyalgia. They found that pain was significantly reduced by land and water-based exercises of slight to moderate intensity when conducted two-three times a week. Exercise also had a positive effect on mood, health-related quality of life, and physical fitness. The authors added that patients should be motivated to continue exercising after seeing the results. (*Arthritis Research & Therapy*, May 10, 2010)

hurt? When? How often? Only two of six types of headaches—tension and migraine—are normally associated with chronic pain.

Tension headaches

Tension headaches are 'featureless,' meaning they are not accompanied by other symptoms. They are usually brought on by fatigue or stress, and those who have them describe a feeling of pressure on both sides of the head. Others experience pain that involves the forehead, scalp, or back of the neck. Tension headaches can be mild, moderate, or severe, but not debilitating. However, occasional episodes can develop into chronic, long-term pain.

Tension headaches can be caused by contractions of the muscles in the head and neck, and expanded blood vessels in the scalp can contribute to the discomfort. They can be triggered by any number of factors, including an argument with a spouse, traffic, job pressures, working at a computer for long periods of time, and poor posture. Arthritis of the cervical facet joints might also be the cause of tension headaches. A lack of exercise appears to be associated with non-migraine headaches.

Tension headaches are usually treated with over-the-counter drugs such as aspirin, Tylenol, or Advil. If you are experiencing them for more than 15 days a month, you have chronic pain and should see a doctor. He or she might prescribe antidepressants, blood pressure medication, or anti-seizure pills.

Migraine headaches

As many as 28 million Americans have migraines, including 25 percent of all adult women, according to the *Journal of the American Medical Association*. Migraines are often misdiagnosed as sinus headaches because the pain is felt across the forehead and the bridge of the nose, just like sinus headaches. Migraine headaches might originate in the protective tissue covering the brain instead of being caused by dilating or constricting blood vessels.

A migraine headache involves recurring episodes (two or more a month) of head pain, plus sensitivity to light and sound. The pain can be accompanied by nausea, vomiting, and neck pain. Ten to 20 percent of the time the person who is about to experience a migraine gets a warning, called an aura. An aura could be a tingling sensation or visual distortion (seeing zigzag lines) that lasts from 10 to 30 minutes.

Migraines are triggered by hormonal changes (caused by menstrual periods or estrogen), diet (alcohol, chocolate, MSG, caffeine, marinated foods), bright lights, strong odors, stress, fatigue, and poor sleep patterns. Researchers believe they are triggered when nerves and blood vessels at the base of the brain stem interact to cause pain. However, biochemical processes in the brain and vascular disease, respectively, are potential migraine causes. In fact, migraines may be associated with heart disease, according to a study published in the February 10, 2010, online issue of *Neurology* (see Box 2-5).

A physician might suggest changes in sleep or eating habits and will probably prescribe medicines to block the pain. Medications called triptans can prevent or treat a migraine. These drugs include sumatriptan (Imitrex), eletriptan (Relpax), and rizatriptan (Maxalt). Injectable triptans have an 80 percent success rate, and triptan tablets are thought to be 60 to 70 percent effective in treating migraines.

A new anti-migraine drug called telcagepant is in the final stages of development, according to a study in the April 2010 issue of *The Lancet*. It represents a new class (not a triptan) that blocks nerve signals and interrupts the metabolic process sufficiently to bring pain relief.

Antidepressants and drugs used to treat high blood pressure (including beta-blockers) also can help prevent migraines. Injecting an anesthetic directly into trigger points in muscles of the neck may eliminate migraine headache symptoms. The treatment may also reduce patients' dependence on drugs, which can sometimes trigger additional headaches.

Some patients may not need prescription drugs to get relief, according to two studies published in the March 2010 issue of the journal *Headache*. Researchers in Thailand concluded that naproxen provided reduced symptoms within two hours, and in a separate study, the makers of Tylenol found that acetaminophen helped 52 percent of subjects as compared to 32 percent in a placebo group (see Box 2-6). In addition, the *Cochrane Systematic Review* (April 13, 2010) reported that a single dose of 900–1000 mg of aspirin may substantially reduce migraine headaches within two hours for more than half the people who take it (see Box 2-7).

There are also data indicating that occipital nerve stimulation (see Chapter 3) is very effective in controlling intractable migraines in some patients.

Herniated disc
Areas most likely affected: lower back, neck
The term 'slipped disc' is often used to refer to disc problems, but it is incorrect—discs do not slip. Instead, some of a disc's soft

---

NEW FINDING

Box 2-6: Naproxen, acetaminophen may provide migraine relief

Two studies show that people with migraine headaches may get relief from over-the-counter drugs such as naproxen and acetaminophen. At Mahidol University in Bangkok, scientists studied 2,168 patients and found that doses of 500-825 milligrams reduced the intensity and pain of headaches within two hours of taking the medication. Researchers at McNeil Consumer Health Care (makers of Tylenol) assigned 37 migraine patients to a group that took either 1,000 mg of Tylenol or a placebo pill. After two hours, 52 percent of the acetaminophen (Tylenol) subjects reported reduced or mild pain, while 32 percent of the placebo group reported diminished symptoms. (*Headache*, March, 2010)

NEW FINDING

Box 2-7: Aspirin may relieve migraine pain in 25-50 percent of patients

A review of 13 studies involving more than 4,000 participants found that severe or moderate migraine pain can be reduced within two hours to no pain in 25 percent of people who take between 900 and 1,000 mg of aspirin. Pain was reduced to no worse than mild pain in 52 percent of the subjects. Researchers also found that aspirin combined with metoclopramide, an antiemetic drug, may be "reasonable therapy" for some acute migraine attacks. (*Cochrane Systematic Review*, April 13, 2010)

material breaks up, bulges into the spinal canal, and puts pressure on a nerve. Anyone can develop a herniated disc, but older adults are especially susceptible.

Herniated disc (lower back)

Lower back and/or leg pain is a commonly reported symptom of a herniated disc. The discomfort, numbness, and tingling can radiate from the buttocks all the way to the toes. The pain worsens with walking, standing and anything that causes intra-abdominal pressure—such as coughing, sneezing, or straining with a bowel movement. Muscle weakness can occur in the affected leg, and muscle spasms are common. The pain resolves itself with or without treatment in up to a third of all cases, but the process can take weeks.

Despite what most people think, a herniated disc in the back is not usually associated with a specific traumatic event. It can occur with a simple activity such as bending over, heavy lifting, or any strenuous activities that generate abdominal pressure. That pressure is transmitted to the disc, often in the L4/L5 vertebrae area (see Box 2-8). Prolonged sitting and repetitive lifting and twisting are risk factors, as is reduced muscle tone caused by a lack of physical activity.

The initial treatment for a herniated disc is rest (including bed rest), ice, plus anti-inflammatory and pain medications. Apply ice for the first 48-72 hours, and then switch to moist heat. There is increasing evidence that mild activity is better than complete or extended periods of bed rest. A type of physical therapy known as the McKenzie Back Program, which involves a series of stretches, is often prescribed to reduce leg pain. It seems to be effective in the short-term, but is no better or worse than other treatments, such as drugs, massage, or strength training.

Longer-term treatment under a physician's care includes medications, epidural steroid injections, and the use of transcutaneous electrical nerve stimulation devices (TENS units) that send electrical impulses into the area to reduce inflammation. Transforaminal epidural steroid injection is a way of delivering the

BOX 2-8: HERNIATED DISC L4/L5

The disc between lumbar vertebrae four and five is often involved in low back pain.

steroid medications around the compressed or irritated nerve root. There is evidence that this technique is effective in improving pain and functionality of patients. It might, in special cases, save patients from having surgery.

Surgery is indicated when the disc clearly will not heal by itself, when there is loss of bowel or bladder function, progressive leg or foot weakness, or an emergency situation. There is a five percent risk of the condition recurring and a greater risk of future back pain, with or without surgery. Remember, not all herniated discs cause pain or require treatment, only if the herniated disc is pinching on one or more nerves in the spinal canal. Your pain physician should be able to determine that.

Prevention is not always possible, but a systematic program of stretching and strengthening is a good place to start. Proper lifting and bending techniques will help you avoid putting your back in a vulnerable position. Warm up before lifting a heavy object, and bend at the knees instead of the waist. Keep your back straight and head forward, maintain a wide stance, test the load before you lift, and hold the load close to your body.

Herniated disc (neck)

Sometimes confused with pain due to bone spurs or arthritis in the area, a herniated disc in the neck is a degenerative condition. It occurs when the material that constitutes a disc breaks up and puts pressure on the surrounding nerves. In most cases, no specific event triggers the herniated disc.

A herniated disc in the neck can cause the following symptoms:

- Neck pain
- Slowed arm reflexes
- Arm numbness, tingling, weakness
- Pain that radiates down the arm
- Numbness of fingers and weakness of hand grip

Elevating the affected arm, bending the elbow, and placing the hand behind the head often relieve the pain. This maneuver eases the pressure on the nerve and enlarges the opening through which the nerve exits the spine. Immediate treatment includes rest, NSAIDs, and physical therapy. You can use a heating pad to relieve muscle spasms.

Long-term relief comes with using a heating pad, taking prescription analgesics and pain relievers, and participating in physical therapy that includes traction. A physician may prescribe the McKenzie neck physical therapy program, which is a systematic series of exercises developed specifically for this type of problem. A six-day course of an oral steroid is an option for severe pain. Epidural steroid injections may be used if the arm pain does not improve with therapy or NSAIDs. Epidural steroids are more effective than oral steroids and are associated with fewer side effects. This approach is much more effective for treating radicular pain secondary to a herniated disc. In many instances it might save patients unnecessary surgery.

Surgery is reserved for persistent arm pain or progressive arm weakness. When it is required, the procedure involves removing the disc (discectomy), or a fragment of the disc, and fusing the adjacent ones.

Irritable bowel syndrome
Areas most likely affected: abdomen, stomach

Approximately 20 percent of Americans will develop irritable bowel syndrome (IBS), one of the most common pain-causing disorders that physicians diagnose. IBS usually starts in early adulthood, and it affects women more often than men.

IBS does not permanently damage the intestines, nor does it lead to serious diseases such as cancer. No one knows what causes IBS. It cannot be traced to any single condition, but research suggests that patients with IBS have a very sensitive colon, which overreacts in response to things that wouldn't bother other people, including food and stress. Evidence also suggests that the immune system might be involved. IBS is often diagnosed when other gastrointestinal conditions have been ruled out. No specific test can confirm its presence.

Most people with IBS can control their symptoms with diet, stress-management techniques, and medications. The most common symptoms are pain (often below the navel), stomach cramps, bloating, constipation, and/or diarrhea. Symptoms of IBS can worsen after eating large meals or fatty foods; taking certain medicines; eating wheat, rye, barley, or chocolate; and drinking milk, alcohol, or caffeine-containing coffee, tea, or soft drinks.

Treatment addresses symptoms, rather than curing IBS. Prescription medications can decrease diarrhea, control colon muscle spasms, and reduce pain. To address the psychological components of IBS, you can try relaxation training, meditation, yoga, exercise, avoiding stressful situations, and getting a good night's sleep.

Osteoporosis
Areas most likely affected: spine, hips, wrists

Osteoporosis causes bones to become thin, fragile, and more likely to break (see Box 2-9). In America, 10 million people have the disease. Osteoporosis is responsible for more than 1.5 million fractures annually, 700,000 of which occur in the spine. Fifty percent of women over the age of 50 are at risk of having a fracture caused by osteoporosis at some point in their lives, but older men who have sustained a minor fracture are as likely to have a subsequent fracture as women. The consequences of untreated osteoporosis and vertebral compression fractures can be very serious.

Osteoporosis has several risk factors, many of which you can control:

Controllable risk factors

- Low estrogen in women
- Low testosterone in men
- Lifetime diet low in calcium/vitamin D
- Anorexia
- Anticonvulsant use
- Inactive lifestyle
- Cigarette smoking
- Excessive alcohol use
- Use of steroids taken orally (patients taking chronic steroids for asthma, rheumatoid arthritis, etc., are at a much higher risk)

Non-controllable risk factors

- Gender (female)
- Age (getting older)
- Race (Caucasians/Asians more susceptible)

Any bone can be affected by osteoporosis, but fractures of the spine and hip are of special concern. A hip fracture almost always requires hospitalization and major surgery. It can impair a person's ability to walk unassisted, and it may cause prolonged or permanent disability, or even death. Spinal fractures also have serious consequences, including height loss, severe back pain, and deformity. Although some people with osteoporosis experience no pain at all, others have intense pain caused not only by the fractures, but also by muscle spasms.

Stress fractures usually take about three months to heal. Pain lasting beyond that period may be considered chronic. The long-term effects of untreated osteoporosis are detrimental. Impaired lung capacity, depression, low self-esteem, and increased risk of fractures are just a few of the complications of osteoporosis.

Osteoporosis is treated by a variety of traditional and alternative therapies, including heat, ice, transcutaneous electrical nerve stimulation (TENS),

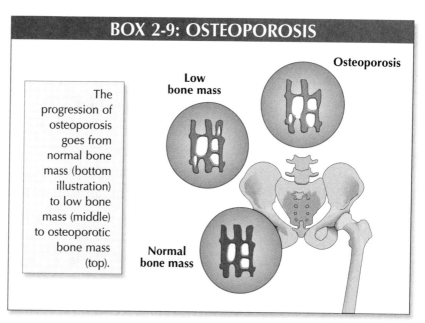

BOX 2-9: OSTEOPOROSIS

The progression of osteoporosis goes from normal bone mass (bottom illustration) to low bone mass (middle) to osteoporotic bone mass (top).

Osteoporosis

Low bone mass

Normal bone mass

exercise, massage, and relaxation. One of the more innovative surgical procedures is called balloon kyphoplasty, which treats the spinal fractures associated with osteoporosis. (See 'Kyphoplasty' in Chapter 3.) The medication strontium ranelate appears to relieve back pain in women who have both osteoporosis and osteoarthritis.

Researchers continue to discover new and interesting ways that have the potential for lowering the risk of osteoporosis. Older men and women who have one or two glasses of beer or wine a day appear to have stronger bones than both non-drinkers and heavy drinkers. However, studies have also shown that even moderate drinking can increase the risk of cancer in postmenopausal women, so the new study should not be taken as a signal for non-drinkers to begin the practice. Benefits should be weighed against risks.

Sciatica
Areas most likely affected: lower back, buttocks, legs

Sciatica is caused by inflammation or pressure on the sciatic nerve, which branches off the spinal cord and extends downward on both sides of the hips, legs, and feet. The most common cause is a herniated disc in the lower back. Symptoms range from mild to severe. The feeling can be one of numbness, tingling, or shooting pain in the lower back that radiates to the buttocks or down the back of one leg. In rare cases, sciatica causes the loss of bladder control. The symptoms may be worse when you cough, sneeze, sit, or do certain types of exercise.

Risk factors for sciatica include:

- Age (30 and over)
- Frequently twisting the back
- Genetic factors
- Diabetes
- An occupation that involves excessive bending, lifting, or driving for long periods of time

With or without treatment, sciatica usually goes away in about six weeks. If it lasts longer, consider making an appointment with a pain management specialist. Good posture, stretching, walking, swimming, lifting objects safely, sleeping on your back or side, and avoiding sitting or standing for long periods of time are ways to prevent sciatica.

Spine surgeons usually recommend a short period of rest followed by exercises to improve flexibility, mobility, and strength in the back. Working with a physical therapist can help chronic pain caused by sciatica. Your doctor may also recommend hot and cold applications. Analgesic and anti-inflammatory drugs such as naproxen, ibuprofen, and aspirin can dull pain and reduce inflammation. Epidural steroid injections are very effective for controlling the leg symptoms.

Shingles
Areas most likely affected: chestwall, waistline, side, face

Nearly one million Americans receive medical care for shingles or its complications each year, according to 2008 report from the Agency for Healthcare Research and Quality. Shingles causes an outbreak of a rash or blisters on the skin. It is a viral disease—the same one that causes chickenpox. After chickenpox heals, the virus becomes dormant in the body, but it can emerge again in about 20 percent of people who have had chickenpox. Those who are at the greatest risk for shingles have a weakened immune system, are over the age of 50, have been ill, are experiencing trauma, and/or are under stress.

The symptoms of shingles often include itching, stabbing, or shooting pains. The skin appears red in the affected area. Other symptoms are fever, chills, headache, and an upset stomach. A rash appears after a few days around the waistline or on one side of the face or trunk.

There is no cure for shingles, but treatment with antiviral medications such as acyclovir (Zovirax), valacyclovir (Valtrex), and famciclovir (Famvir) can help ease the pain and discomfort and reduce the duration of symptoms. A vaccine called Zostavax can help prevent shingles in adults 60 and older, and can reduce nerve pain when shingles does occur. Oxycodone can be an effective treatment for the pain caused by shingles.

A painful complication of shingles is called postherpetic neuralgia (PHN).

Postherpetic neuralgia

Even after the blisters of shingles heal, the nerve pain can remain. Although this pain gradually fades, it can persist for years.

Not everyone who has shingles develops postherpetic neuralgia, but older people are at high risk. The older you are when you first get shingles, the more likely you are to develop PHN. Half of people over the age of 60 who get shingles develop PHN, while 75 percent of those over 70 get the condition.

The primary symptom of PHN is severe unilateral pain that can lead to insomnia, weight loss, and depression. More specifically, symptoms include:

- Sharp, jabbing, burning, deep, or aching pain
- Unusual sensitivity to touch and temperature change
- Itching or numbness

The shingles vaccine can help prevent the disease (and thus its complications) in adults over 60, and it can relieve the pain of postherpetic neuralgia if the disease does occur. Treatment for PHN includes skin patches containing Lidocaine, antidepressants, anticonvulsants, painkillers, and transcutaneous electrical nerve stimulation (TENS). Some patients get relief from one or more of those treatments, but most people continue to have some pain. Studies show that aggressive treatment of acute phase 'shingles' with nerve blocks may decrease the chances of developing PHN. Researchers also have found that treatment with intravenous and oral antiviral medications, such as acyclovir, may reduce nerve pain. Newer anti-neuropathic pain agents such as pregabalin (Lyrica) are very effective in treating PHN, with minimal side effects.

Spinal stenosis
Areas most likely affected: back and neck

Stenosis is a narrowing of the spinal canal that pinches the spinal cord and nerves. Potential causes are aging, heredity, tumors, trauma, and repeated back surgery. The result is pain in the lower back and legs that can be aggravated by walking and standing. The condition is characterized by numbness, tingling, hot or cold sensations, weakness, or leg fatigue. Some people feel more clumsy than usual or have falls. Because other conditions can also cause these symptoms, it's important to see your doctor for a full evaluation.

Leaning forward slightly while you're walking, and lying down with your knees drawn to your chest can temporarily relieve the symptoms of spinal stenosis. For more long-term symptom relief, try anti-inflammatory medicines such as aspirin and ibuprofen, and rest the affected area. Cleveland Clinic's Department of Pain Management researchers, upon review of hundreds of cases of spinal stenosis, found that epidural steroid injections combined with physical therapy resulted in significant pain relief. Increased walking distance and standing time are two important features that indicate the success of the treatment.

Surgery to relieve pressure on the affected nerves previously has been a treatment of last resort, but surgery appears to be better than nonsurgical treatments for the condition. Two minimally-invasive procedures—

X-STOP and MILD—are examples. X-STOP maintains space between vertebrae to prevent pressure, and MILD uses x-ray guidance to remove some bone and soft tissue that decreases the size of the spinal canal without the need for laminectory surgery. Initial results at Cleveland Clinic Pain Management have been very encouraging. See Chapter 3 for more information.

Doctors will encourage you to gradually resume physical activities such as bicycling, extension exercises, water exercises, or swimming, as you feel able. If you're overweight, losing the extra weight will reduce the load on your spine and help relieve your pain. You should be able to walk further and stand for longer periods of time once your symptoms have improved.

TMD/TMJ
(temporomandibular joint disorders)
Areas most likely affected: jaw, head, ear, face

TMJ is usually associated with pain in the jaw. Physicians are more likely to use the acronym TMD, which stands for temporomandibular disorders—a group of symptoms that affect the joints connecting the lower jaw to the skull. The matching joints are located on each side of the head directly in front of your ears. TMJ refers to the joint, but is often used to describe any disorder or symptom in this region. Symptoms of TMD/TMJ include:

- Inability to open the mouth
- Pain in the jaw, face, or ears
- Headaches
- Toothaches

TMJ symptoms can be caused by clenching and grinding the teeth, poor head and shoulder posture, the inability to relax, and lack of sleep. Arthritis, fractures, joint degeneration, or structural abnormalities can also result in contracted muscles and pinched nerves in the jaw, head, and neck.

Diagnosing and treating TMJ might require a team of specialists, including a primary care physician, dentist, and ear-nose-throat (ENT) doctor. Treatment ranges from mouth guards to massage, as well as moist heat, cold applications, and exercises to help you relax your jaw. More aggressive therapy involves muscle relaxants, NSAIDs, orthodontics, and, very rarely, reconstructive surgery. TMJ pain tends to be cyclical; it can go away temporarily and then return in the future.

Trigeminal neuralgia
Areas most likely affected: head, face, jaws

Trigeminal neuralgia (TN) affects one of the largest nerves in the head. The trigeminal nerve carries impulses of touch, pain, pressure, and temperature to the brain from the face, jaw, gums, forehead, and around the eyes. TN occurs when a blood vessel puts pressure on the nerve. The distinguishing characteristic is a sudden, electric-shock-like pain on one side of the jaw or cheek lasting for up to a couple of minutes. Attacks may occur one after the other, and can be triggered by talking, brushing the teeth, touching the face, chewing, swallowing, or even by a breeze that touches the face. Episodes can last for months and then disappear for years. The disorder is more common in women than in men and mostly affects people over the age of 50.

Treatment for TN typically includes anticonvulsant medications. One of those drugs, pregabalin, has been shown to be an effective treatment for TN. Radiofrequency ablation of the trigeminal ganglion should be considered before surgery. If medication and radiofrequency ablation fails to relieve pain, surgery may be recommended. Gamma knife radiosurgery (GKRS) is a promising treatment for trigeminal neuralgia. GKRS is a non-invasive, outpatient treatment that aims narrow beams of radioactive cobalt at the trigeminal nerve. Ninety percent of patients have significant pain relief within an average of four weeks after GKRS, and 80 percent have a significant improvement in their quality of life.

Trigger points
Areas most likely affected: upper and lower back, neck, and hips

Trigger points—extremely tight, sensitive, and localized areas of muscle spasm that occur most often in the upper back, neck, and lower lumbar muscles—are relatively common among people who engage in repetitive-motion activities. Symptoms such as tightness, extreme sensitivity to pressure, and restricted range of motion, come and go. The exact cause of trigger points is unknown, but they may be instigated by staying in one position too long, overusing the muscles in the affected area, and stress.

Typical treatment (other than pain medication) is performed by a physical therapist or massage therapist, who puts direct, sustained pressure on the sensitive part of the muscle to reduce tightness and pain. Just a few minutes of pressure can provide relief for hours or even days. ■

3 TRADITIONAL PAIN MANAGEMENT

Drugs play an important role in the treatment of chronic pain, but physicians at the Cleveland Clinic understand that chronic pain patients may need more than painkillers. Patients need a wide range of treatments in varying disciplines such as physical and occupational therapy, individual and group therapy, stress management, and cognitive behavioral therapy. Cognitive behavioral therapy (to reduce negative thoughts and behaviors) may be effective in treating chronic back pain, according to a study in the February 26, 2010, edition of *The Lancet* (see Box 3-1).

Minimally-invasive treatments may sometimes include sympathetic or somatic nerve blocks, radiofrequency or cryoblation, intrathecal drug pumps, and spinal cord stimulation. Surgery is another option for patients with more complicated issues.

"Collaborative Care Intervention" which includes education, monitoring symptoms, and providing feedback to the primary care physician is now considered to be more effective than traditional pain management strategies.

Here are some potential options for treating chronic pain:

- Cold applications (cryotherapy)
- Heat applications (thermotherapy)
- Medications (nine drug groups)
- Bioelectric treatment
- TENS (transcutaneous electrical nerve stimulation)
- PENS (percutaneous electrical nerve stimulation)
- OCS (occipital nerve stimulation)
- Nerve blocks
- Spinal cord stimulation
- Deep brain stimulation
- Drug infusion pumps
- Surgery (13 procedures)

Cold applications (cryotherapy)

Cold applications (cryotherapy) can be used as a temporary solution for a long-term problem. The technique decreases temperature, inflammation, rate of metabolic activity, circulation, muscle spasms, and pain. It shrinks blood vessels and, in doing so, minimizes bleeding and swelling. In medical terms, ice reduces pain because it reduces nerve end sensitivity. In lay terms, ice deadens the pain in that area.

If you have aggravated an old injury, the general rule is to use ice for the first 48-72 hours or until the swelling subsides. At first the ice will feel uncomfortably cold. Then you'll feel a burning sensation, followed by an aching feeling, and finally, numbness. Ice can temporarily relieve pain almost any time. Another guideline: use ice if pain limits your motion, and use heat if stiffness limits your motion.

Apply ice for 10- to 30-minute periods, separated by at least an hour between applications. The duration of applications should also vary with the area of the body being iced. Tissues, muscles, and structures that lie close to the surface of the skin or have little surrounding body fat require less icing time than those that lie deeper in the body.

The most common method of icing is to place a wet towel over the affected area, with an ice bag positioned on top of the towel. Use a bandage to keep the bag in place. Chemical ice bags are acceptable and have various degrees of effectiveness, but don't place them directly against the skin and be careful not to apply so much pressure that the bag breaks. An ice massage is another alternative, and it can cool muscle tissue faster than an ice bag. For an ice massage, freeze water in a paper or Styrofoam cup, turn the cup upside down, and peel the paper away as the ice melts against your skin. Keep a towel handy to absorb the melting ice water. If the area is small enough, another option is to immerse it in an ice bucket for five to 10 minutes. When using ice, don't hold the ice for more than a few minutes on a small area, avoid using it on blisters or open wounds, and don't ice before exercising.

People who are overly sensitive to cold won't be able to tolerate ice applications long enough for them to be effective. Also, those with blood vessels near the surface of the skin and anyone who has a condition called Raynaud's phenomenon should not use ice. If you have diabetes or any other condition that diminishes blood flow, check with your doctor before applying ice packs.

Heat applications (thermotherapy)

Heat applications (thermotherapy) increase the flow of blood, nutrients, and oxygen to affected areas of the body. Applying heat can also relieve pain by relaxing the muscles, producing a sedative effect, and decreasing muscle tension.

Heat effectively masks some cases of chronic pain, but it has not been proven to cure it and should not be considered a long-term solution. Also, the increased flow of blood can cause swelling in the area, which in some people may be fueling their pain in the first place. However, heat may offer relief from conditions such as back and neck pain, and osteoarthritis. Heat therapy appears to improve osteoarthritis-related knee pain, stiffness, and function.

Use heat for chronic pain whenever you think it will ease your pain, as long as you have your doctor's permission. Wet heat can be more effective because it penetrates deeper than dry heat. A hydrocollator is a heating pad that applies moist heat to superficial and subcutaneous (just below the surface) tissues. Do not apply heat to bare skin immediately after an injury.

Medications

A number of medications are approved by the Food and Drug Administration (FDA) for managing pain. Some have been in use for many years, whereas others are more recent.

Acetaminophen

Acetaminophen (found in Tylenol, Datril, and several forms of Excedrin) is generally safe and effective for relieving pain (although not inflammation), especially for osteoarthritis of the hip and knee. It is also as effective as naproxen and ibuprofen in relieving lower back pain. Although this drug has little risk if used according to directions, taking too much too often can cause liver damage and even death. Men who regularly take acetaminophen and other common pain relievers may have an increased risk of high blood pressure. Overdoses of acetaminophen account for 40-50 percent of all acute liver failure cases each year in the United States. Before taking acetaminophen, tell your doctor if you have had liver disease, or if you drink alcohol on a regular basis. Also, read the labels of all your medications to find out if they contain acetaminophen. Per a new FDA warning, it is advisable NOT to exceed 2,000 mg/day of acetaminophen.

Antidepressants

Several painful conditions respond to antidepressants (see Box 3-2), a group of drugs that works by increasing the concentration of certain chemical messengers (neurotransmitters) in the brain, some of which directly relieve pain. The primary role of antidepressants is to treat depression, which is closely intertwined with pain. Chronic pain can lead to depression, and depression can magnify the awareness of pain.

Low-dose tricyclic antidepressants (TCAs) such as amitriptyline, imipramine (Tofranil), and desipramine (Norpramine) have been used for some time in the treatment of pain related to nerve damage (neuropathic pain).

BOX 3-2

Types of pain that may respond to antidepressants

- Central pain (after a stroke)
- Fibromyalgia
- Irritable bowel syndrome
- Postherpetic neuralgia
- Sympathetic dystrophy
- Diabetic neuropathy
- Migraine and tension headaches
- Phantom limb pain
- Stump/neuroma pain
- Peripheral neuropathy caused by chemotherapy

The relatively low doses of TCAs that are used to treat pain have fewer side effects (like sedation and dry mouth) than the high-dose TCAs used to treat depression. Venlafaxine (Effexor) is a newer antidepressant (not a trycyclic) that has proven to be effective in treating lower back pain, osteoarthritis, and rheumatoid arthritis. Duloxetine HCI (Cymbalta) has recently shown promise in reducing chronic lower back pain, according to data presented at the 2010 meeting of the American Academy of Pain Medicine (see Box 3-3).

Some antidepressants may be as effective as most opioids for improving patients' chronic pain and ability to function. In addition to antidepressants, anti-anxiety drugs also act as muscle relaxants and are occasionally used as pain relievers.

Antidepressants can have unpleasant side effects, such as sedation, nausea, weight gain, sexual problems, dry mouth, and blurred vision. Daily use of selective serotonin reuptake inhibitors (SSRIs) may significantly increase the risk of fractures.

Aspirin

Aspirin is considered one of the most effective methods of relieving pain, but it carries side effects, most notably stomach-lining irritation and blood thinning. Avoid the use of aspirin when you have used alcohol or taken blood thinners, corticosteroids, medications for hypertension or diabetes, methotrexate, or probenecid. Also avoid taking aspirin together with ibuprofen. A 2007 study revealed that using the two drugs together can increase the risk for heart attack, and can negate the cardio-preventive benefits of daily aspirin therapy. The chart on this page lists four over-the-counter medications, the conditions they best treat, and possible side effects (see Box 3-4).

Cox-2 inhibitors

COX-2 inhibitors reduce inflammation without the stomach irritation and bleeding risks associated with the non-steroidal anti-inflammatory agents, but an association exists between this group of drugs and heart problems, especially in high-risk patients. Celebrex is the only COX-2 inhibitor still available (albeit with a "Black Box" warning indicating its risks), but physicians are prescribing the drug with caution.

BOX 3-4: OVER-THE COUNTER PAIN MEDICATION

MEDICATION	BEST TO TREAT	POSSIBLE SIDE EFFECTS
ASPIRIN	migraines, fever, moderate pain	bleeding, stomach irritation
IBUPROFEN	muscle pain, headache, minor pain	minor bleeding, nausea
ACETAMINOPHEN	fever, headache, minor pain	liver toxicity in high doses
NAPROXEN	arthritis pain	dizziness, cold symptoms, gastrointestinal distress

Nonsteroidal anti-inflammatory drugs (NSAIDs)

Nonsteroidal anti-inflammatory drugs (NSAIDs) such as ibuprofen (Motrin, Advil) and naproxen (Naprosyn) are commonly used for arthritis, headaches, and other types of pain. They can, however, cause intestinal tract irritation and bleeding, and some NSAIDs and NSAID doses present a greater threat than others, according to new research published in the February 22, 2010, issue of *Arthritis & Rheumatism* (see Box 3-5).

Taking more than one type of NSAID during the same period of time (one month, for example) has a negative effect on both physical and mental health, and that multiple use should be avoided.

Opioids

Opioids (also called narcotics) are one of the most prescribed and controversial of all the pain-relieving drugs. Natural opioids are derived from the opium poppy, but synthetic opioids can be produced in the laboratory. Examples of generic opioids are codeine and morphine; trade names include Dilaudid, Demerol, and OxyContin. All are effective in relieving both acute and chronic pain, but they produce side effects, including drowsiness, dizziness, and constipation.

Opioids are controversial because they carry the potential for physical and psychological dependence. Some doctors are hesitant to prescribe them, both for medical and legal reasons, even though several studies have shown that the probability of addiction among chronic pain patients who do not have a history of substance abuse is low. A University of Wisconsin research team found 3.9 percent of chronic pain patients abuse opioids. While the rate is four times higher than abuse in the general population, it is still low. A separate study found that less than three percent of patients with no history of drug abuse who are prescribed opioids for chronic pain will show signs of possible drug abuse or dependence. Proponents of opioids argue that withholding them causes unnecessary pain, that side effects can be managed, and that the risk of addiction is overstated.

Drugs are being developed that would counteract the abuse potential of narcotics. An opioid antagonist drug could be combined with a painkilling narcotic but not be activated unless the patient tried to take too much of the narcotic or to take it too often.

To avoid abuse and diversion of opioids, the Department of Pain Management at Cleveland Clinic uses a medication agreement signed by the physician and patient to regulate the use, prescription, and dispensing of opioids.

Opioids also raise the risk of bone fractures in older adults, according to a study in the January 5, 2010, online issue of the *Journal of General Internal*

NEW FINDING

Box 3-5: Not all NSAIDs equal in risk of internal bleeding

The risk of bleeding while on non-steroidal anti-inflammatory drugs (NSAIDs) increases with age, with the type of pain-killing drug, and with the amount taken. Spanish researchers analyzed the results of nine studies over a period of nine years to discover that doses of 1,200-2,400 mg of ibuprofen daily increased bleeding by five times more than doses of up to 1,200 mg. Prescription-level ibuprofen (not sold over the counter) also increased the risk of gastrointestinal bleeding more than low-dose non-prescription NSAIDs. For those not taking prescription NSAIDs, the risk of bleeding remains low — about one-tenth of one percent. *(Arthritis & Rheumatism, online February 22, 2010)*

Medicine (see Box 3-6). The annual fracture rate increased in the over-60 age group increased from four to 10 percent among those taking opioid drugs.

Steroids

Steroids are effective in treating inflammation and pain, as well as the underlying causes of pain such as lupus and rheumatoid arthritis. They are usually prescribed for short periods of time because they produce side effects such as depression and osteoporosis, and they can become less effective over time.

Topical pain relievers

Topical pain relievers come in creams, sprays, patches, and rubs. Some of them, such as lidocaine (Lidoderm), fentanyl (Duragesic), and Flector Patch (a NSAID that is used transdermally), are applied to the skin directly or through 'pain patches.' When the medication is absorbed into the skin, it blocks the pain signals to the brain.

EMLA cream is a topical anesthetic containing lidocaine and prilocaine. It is applied before certain medical procedures and its effects can last for up to three hours under a dressing, and for one to two hours after the cream is removed.

Capsaicin, which comes from the seeds of chili peppers, is used to treat pain associated with arthritis, shingles, and diabetes, among other conditions. It can provide temporary relief over long periods of time, but can irritate the skin and produce a burning sensation in the first few weeks of use. You may have to use capsaicin for three to four weeks to determine whether it is effective. Capsaicin works by stimulating nerve ending receptors, which send a message to the brain that generates the sensation of pain and allows calcium to enter the cells until the receptors shut down.

Other drugs

Ziconotide (Prialt) and pregabalin (Lyrica) are relatively new drugs used for managing pain. Prialt belongs to a class of drugs known as N-type calcium channel blockers. It is administered by infusion directly into the spinal fluid, and is believed to target and block the channels that transmit pain signals. It is a synthetic non-narcotic drug and does not cause addiction. It is very effective for neuropathic pain, however, slow titration (giving the lowest effective amount) of the dose is highly recommended to avoid serious side effects. Lyrica comes in capsule form and is used for managing pain associated with diabetic peripheral neuropathy and postherpetic neuralgia. It is the first treatment approved by the FDA for both conditions. Side effects of

Lyrica include dizziness, drowsiness, dry mouth, and blurred vision. Pain relief lasts for up to 12 weeks. Studies showed Lyrica is effective in cases of neuropathic pain that failed to respond to other drugs such as Neurontin. Recently, pregabalin has been approved by the FDA to treat fibromyalgia.

Rituximab (Rituxan), abatacept (Orencia), and tocilizumab (Actemra) are relatively new drugs used for patients with rheumatoid arthritis. All three drugs reduce the symptoms of rheumatoid arthritis, improve patients' physical function, and slow the progression of joint damage. About half of patients saw improvements in their symptoms after taking Orencia or Actemra with the widely used RA drug, methotrexate. Rituxan and Orencia have been approved for RA treatment, but in September of 2008 the FDA delayed its approval for Actemra and requested more information from the manufacturer.

Zoledronic acid (Reclast) has been approved by the FDA as a single-dose treatment for postmenopausal osteoporosis, as well as a bone condition known as Paget's disease.

For a comprehensive report on medications used to treat chronic pain, visit the American Chronic Pain Association's web site (www.theacpa.org) and download the *ACPA Consumer Guide to Pain Medication & Treatment, 2009 Edition.*

Some topical medications contain trolamine salicylate, which is similar to aspirin. These medications have trade names like Aspercreme and Sportscreme, and appear to be safe, but there is little evidence that they are effective for chronic pain. Others, like Ben-Gay and Icy Hot, stimulate sensory receptors and may distract you from mild muscle or joint soreness, but they are also not likely to help relieve chronic pain.

Bioelectric treatment

Bioelectric treatment involves a precise dose of bioelectric currents administered through electrodes placed on the skin. These currents cause a biological change and interrupt pain signals. This procedure can treat chronic and acute pain conditions, including arthritis, complex regional pain syndrome, back pain, muscle pain, and headaches. Bioelectric therapy also prompts the body to produce endorphins, which are like natural pain relievers. Bioelectric treatment is not recommended for people who have a pacemaker, are pregnant, have blood clots in the arms or legs, or have a bacterial infection.

Transcutaneous electrical nerve stimulation (TENS)

Transcutaneous electrical nerve stimulation (TENS) reduces the sensation of pain. It consists of a portable, battery-powered unit, with

Box 3-7: TENS not recommended for long-term low-back pain

Transcutaneous electronic nerve stimulation is not recommended for pain in the lower back, according to updated guidelines issued by the American Academy of Neurology. The strongest evidence in a review of studies showed that "there is no benefit for people using TENS for chronic low-back pain that has lasted three months or longer." However, the guidelines did say that TENS may be effective in treating diabetic nerve pain, also called diabetic neuropathy. People who are using TENS for back pain should discuss it with their physicians. The guidelines represent another in a series of conflicting reports on the therapeutic use of TENS. (Neurology, December 30, 2009)

electrical leads that are attached to the skin over the painful area. TENS units are usually used in clinical settings by physical therapists, but patients can purchase them for home use with a doctor's prescription. A doctor, nurse, or therapist should teach you how to use it, and you'll need someone at home to help position the leads, especially if you are going to use them on your back.

TENS sends an electrical current through the skin that lasts a fraction of a second, followed by a pause, and the next wave of current. It can be adjusted to deliver intermittent waves. Your doctor or therapist will prescribe the appropriate session length. Normally, you would use a TENS unit for 15 to 30 minutes, several times a day, but you can turn it on or off as needed to control your pain.

How TENS therapy works is unknown. It may stimulate the production of substances in the body that diminish pain. Another possibility is simply that the electrical waves distract you from your pain. The current generates enough heat to relieve stiffness and improve mobility, and is often used for physical therapy in combination with other treatments.

In a treatment called iontophoresis, TENS delivers topical steroid medication through the skin to treat acute episodes of pain. The mild current causes the medication to move into inflamed, soft tissue.

TENS therapy does not work for everyone. In December of 2009, the American Academy of Neurology issued new guidelines stating that TENS is not recommended to treat chronic lower back pain that has persisted for three months or longer because it is not effective (see Box 3-7).

Arrange for a trial period before buying a unit or committing to rent one for an extended period of time.

Some insurance carriers cover the cost (which can be several hundred dollars); others do not. Under certain circumstances, Medicare may cover TENS units. One warning: if you use a pacemaker, do not try TENS. The current could disrupt your pacemaker's operation.

Percutaneous electrical nerve stimulation (PENS)

Percutaneous electrical nerve stimulation (PENS) involves inserting very thin needles into the skin and then sending electrical impulses through the needles to the affected nerves. PENS is usually reserved for patients who get no pain relief from transcutaneous electrical nerve stimulation (TENS), possibly due to scar tissue or fat tissue that prevents the conduction of electrical impulses.

Although they appear similar, PENS is not like acupuncture, in which the needles are placed at strategic points around the body that correlate to the flow of energy. The placement of needles in PENS is determined by their proximity to the area of pain.

Before undergoing PENS, you will be evaluated by a pain management team. You might have a trial placement of the needles to see if they work.

PENS has been shown to be effective in treating chronic lower back pain.

Occipital nerve stimulation (ONS)

An electronic device about the size of a credit card could give chronic headache sufferers a fresh perspective on life (see Box 3-8). Headache specialists are conducting trials using the occipital nerve stimulator (ONS) to help patients with migraine and other types of headache. The stimulator is a small electrical device that is inserted under the skin. Leads from the stimulator are connected to specific nerves that are involved in headache pain. At the first sign of a headache, the patient activates the device, which electrically stimulates the nerve. The brain responds to the electrical stimulation, and the headache pain is blocked. The Department of Pain Management at the Cleveland Clinic shared a multi-center study to evaluate the effectiveness of ONS in treating migraine headaches. Results of the study are very promising and it will be published in a major medical journal in the very near future.

Many patients suffer from pain outside of the area treated by ONS. Peripheral nerve stimulation is promising for intractable headaches in certain patients.

A nerve stimulation device that is the size of a matchstick and that is implanted near the occipital nerve in the back of the neck has been shown to significantly reduce disabling headaches.

Nerve blocks

'Nerve block' is a general term referring to the injection of a local anesthetic or other substance around or near a nerve, nerve network, or pain-sensitive trigger point. Nerve blocks can help those who suffer from many causes of chronic pain, including lower back and neck pain, sciatica and spinal stenosis, complex regional pain syndrome (CRPS), peripheral vascular disease, shingles, myofascial pain syndrome, and cancer pain.

Nerve blocks (also known as regional anesthesia) relieve pain by interrupting pain pathways and preventing pain messages from reaching the brain. In addition to anesthetics, there are various other nerve-block methods. Corticosteroids treat an area of inflammation, such as a herniated disc,

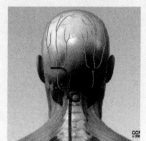

BOX 3-8

OCCIPITAL NERVE STIMULATION

In occipital nerve stimulation, leads to an electrical device are positioned across the occipital nerves. When prompted by the patient, the leads are activated and the brain responds by blocking the headache pain.

nerve entrapment, or a pain trigger point. Opioids (such as morphine) can be infused into the area surrounding the spinal cord to control pain in certain areas of the body. Alcohol or phenol may be used to destroy selective nervous tissues, as might cryoanalgesia (freezing) and radiofrequency (heat).

Nerve blocks can take the form of a single injection or continuous infusion. Pain relief can last from several hours to several months. A slow-release injectable nerve block can provide relief from chronic pain for several months.

The real value of nerve blocks in the management of chronic pain is to provide pain relief for certain periods of time. Such periods of pain relief are utilized to allow rehabilitation. Therefore, in chronic pain, it is a tool to facilitate rehabilitation. Getting nerve blocks without rehabilitation is like using bandages that do not provide long-term benefits.

In many cases, nerve blocks are performed in conjunction with a rehabilitation program. For example, the period of pain relief might be long enough so that a patient can strengthen the muscles of an area through an exercise program. The increased muscle strength could, in turn, relieve or eliminate the symptoms.

Ultrasound imaging might address the problem of finding the proper location to administer a nerve block. Ultrasound guides the physician to peripheral nerves and adjacent structures and tracks the needle movement in real time. Although ultrasound imaging is not standard practice at this time, many anesthesiologists think it will become a valuable part of the nerve block procedure.

No single treatment is guaranteed to produce complete pain relief. Nerve blocks are effective for temporary pain control in some cases; however, they are of limited use for the short-term relief of lower back pain and of no use for long-term relief. Even when they are recommended, nerve blocks should be considered as just one part of a total pain management program.

Nerve blocks have potential side effects. In rare cases, people have allergic reactions to the local anesthetics used in them. Steroids used in nerve blocks can cause fluid retention, increased appetite, blood pressure and blood sugar fluctuations, and mood swings. Morphine and its derivatives can cause constipation, urinary retention, itching, nausea, and vomiting. The destruction of nerve tissue can lead to the partial loss of muscle and nerve functions.

Patients who are on anti-blood clotting therapy with heparin, warfarin (Coumadin), or clopidogrel bisulfate (Plavix), which increase the risk of bleeding, should not have a nerve block. In addition, you should not have a nerve block if there is an active infection around an area where the nerve block is to be given.

Spinal cord stimulation (SCS)

Spinal cord stimulation uses a tiny implanted generator to stimulate the spinal cord, in order to treat a variety of painful conditions and improve circulation (see Box 3-9). Lower back and leg pain or numbness are two of the conditions in which SCS might be an option, but the technique is not for everyone.

The most likely candidates for spinal cord stimulation have had failed spinal surgery; severe nerve-related pain or numbness caused by sciatica; or other chronic pain conditions such as regional pain syndrome, peripheral vascular disease, or angina pain (in patients who are not candidates for bypass surgery).

To undergo spinal cord stimulation, you cannot have an untreated drug addiction or a pacemaker, and a psychological evaluation is a prerequisite. In one study, approximately 60 percent of people who had spinal cord stimulation reported pain reduction or relief one to two years after the procedure. Another study found that the sooner the stimulator is implanted following failed back surgery, the better the chances of pain relief become. Researchers at Cleveland Clinic found that spinal cord stimulation resulted in lower scores on a pain-perception scale and reduced the use of opioids among patients with chronic pelvic pain.

SCS has several advantages. The device is totally implanted and allows you to resume more daily activities than other treatment methods. You can have a trial before agreeing to have a system implanted. You can adjust the device or turn it off. Finally, a physician can remove the device at your request. Also, researchers at the Pain Management Department at the Cleveland Clinic have found that in properly selected patients, SCS is associated with significant healthcare utilization savings.

Typical risks associated with surgery, including bleeding, infection, and allergic reactions, accompany SCS. Following implantation, risks include mechanical malfunctions, stimulation of the wrong location, and infection. Also, be aware that the device can set off metal detectors, and you are not

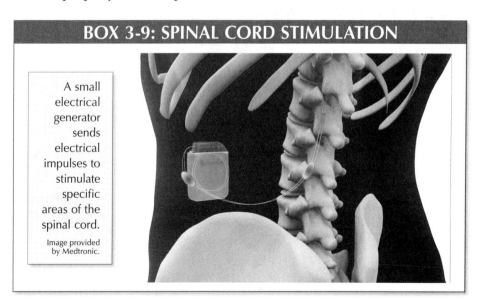

BOX 3-9: SPINAL CORD STIMULATION

A small electrical generator sends electrical impulses to stimulate specific areas of the spinal cord.

Image provided by Medtronic.

supposed to drive while it is on. Finally, you could develop a tolerance to the electrical stimulation, making it less effective over time. In that case, the device will need to be reprogrammed.

In the past, patients needed surgery every one to five years to replace the stimulator's batteries. Now, neurostimulators with rechargeable batteries reduce the need for repeat surgeries, allowing the physician to concentrate on managing the patient instead of managing the battery. Rechargeable batteries can last for up to nine years.

Deep brain stimulation

Deep brain (intracerebral) stimulation (DBS) is an extremely aggressive method of pain control that involves surgically stimulating the brain. It is used for a limited number of conditions, including severe pain, cancer pain, and pain related to nerve damage (neuropathic pain). With DNS, electrodes are surgically implanted in the brain. The patient determines the frequency and extent of stimulation, operating a transmitter that sends signals to a receiver connected to the electrodes (which are located under the skin). This type of analgesia is costly and risky. Nevertheless, patients who have used this technique report that their pain seems to disappear. Other senses are not affected, and there is none of the mental confusion often associated with opioid drug therapy. Deep brain stimulation also might have the potential to reduce cluster headaches.

Drug infusion pumps

A drug infusion pump, pain pump, or medication pump is a device that administers medication directly into the spinal fluid or into the epidural space that surrounds the spinal cord (see Box 3-10). A wide variety of medications or combination of medications can be delivered through the pump. For example, morphine or other narcotics can be used in the pump as painkillers, and muscle relaxers such as baclofen (Lioresal) can be infused to control muscle spasms.

The pain pump is an option when other methods have not effectively relieved chronic pain, or when pain medications taken by other means cause side effects. A doctor determines the exact dosage and frequency of drug

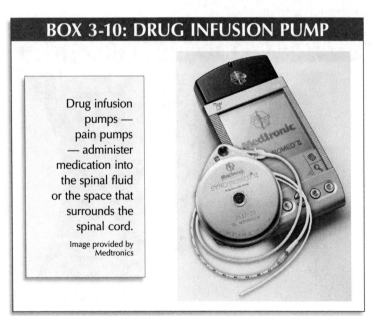

BOX 3-10: DRUG INFUSION PUMP

Drug infusion pumps — pain pumps — administer medication into the spinal fluid or the space that surrounds the spinal cord.

Image provided by Medtronics

infusion delivery. A newer version of the pain pump can enable patients to provide themselves with a breakthrough dose, if needed.

The pump is placed under the skin of the abdomen and attached to a small tube. This technique requires much less medication than other delivery methods because it delivers medicine directly to the spinal cord. As little as 1/300 of the amount of morphine is needed when compared to taking it orally. Since the body is not flooded with medication, the side effects of sedation are much less profound. When the pump is close to being empty, it can be refilled by injecting the medication through the skin and into the reservoir of the pump. Your pain management physician can remove the pump at any time.

Before you make a decision to use a drug pump on a long-term basis, your doctor should conduct a trial with a temporary external pump for at least a few days. A successful trial ought to reduce your existing level of pain by at least half, as well as improve your functional abilities. The drug pump can lessen chronic pain in failed back surgery syndrome, cancer, chronic pancreatitis, and several conditions affecting the nervous system. Pumps can also treat muscle spasms and pain associated with multiple sclerosis, stroke, brain injury, spinal cord injury, and cerebral palsy.

Medication pumps have risks, but most are rare. The trial period should determine whether you are going to develop problems such as a poor response to medications, urinary retention, or allergic reactions. Other long-term complications, although rare, include headaches, spinal cord injury, paralysis, mechanical failure, and infection. Signs of infection include fever, increased pain, drainage, redness, swelling, or an unpleasant odor.

Newer models of the pump have the capability to allow patients to self-administer small doses of pain medicine as needed within the safety limits outlined by the treating physician.

Pumps emit a beeping signal to let you know when a problem occurs, when to change the unit, or when to refill the supply of medicine. The battery and unit can last for three to five years, depending upon the amount of medication delivered. When the battery goes, so does the pump, and it's time for a new one. It is essential to have regular follow-up visits with your physician when using a drug infusion pump. It is advisable not to wait to hear the beep before refilling the pump. You can develop withdrawal symptoms if you allow the pump to run dry.

Surgical options

Surgery is necessary for only a fraction of chronic pain patients. It is usually a last resort, and it doesn't have an especially good success record. Unless surgery can correct an obvious structural or mechanical problem, your doctor is not likely to recommend it until all other treatments have failed.

Minimally-invasive endoscopic spinal surgery

Endoscopic surgery refers to surgical techniques that use very small video cameras and instruments, which are passed through small incisions (less than 2 cm) into the chest, abdominal, or joint cavity. Because the size of the incisions is smaller, the recovery from endoscopic surgery is much quicker than from traditional open surgery. There is also less pain and reduced damage to the surrounding tissues.

Endoscopic techniques have been used for several decades, but were in the past used exclusively for diagnostic purposes. Today, these techniques are commonly used in the treatment of spinal disorders. In certain cases of degenerative disc disease, scoliosis, kyphosis, spinal column tumors, infection, fractures, and herniated discs, endoscopic techniques may speed recovery, minimize post-operative pain and improve the final outcome. Surgery that once required three to six months of recovery now only requires three to six weeks. Not every patient is a candidate for endoscopic spinal surgery. To see if endoscopic treatment is appropriate for your condition, you must be fully evaluated by a knowledgeable and experienced surgeon.

Artificial discs

The FDA has approved a plastic and steel device that can replace a damaged disc in the spinal column of some patients. The damaged disc is removed and an artificial core that floats between two metal plates is put in its place. The disc could be an alternative for some of the 200,000 Americans who undergo spinal fusion surgery each year. Spinal fusion is an operation in which bone is grafted onto the spine, creating a solid union between two or more vertebrae. Although spinal fusion surgery relieves pain, it can restrict mobility. Research found that people with the artificial disc did as well after the procedure as those who had spinal fusion, and individuals with the artificial disc were able to maintain better neck motion than those with spinal fusion. Although the American Academy of Orthopaedic Surgeons has expressed concern about the technically demanding nature of the artificial disc procedure, the number of patients who choose this option is increasing.

Back surgery

Even though we often associate surgery with chronic back pain, only one percent of patients require it. Back surgery typically has two purposes:

decompression, for patients who have a disc or bone pressing on a nerve; and stabilization, which stabilizes and strengthens a weak area in the spine.

Among the surgical options for the back are discectomy, microdiscectomy, and percutaneous disc removal, all of which remove all or part of a protruding disc. Laser disc compression, also called nucleoplasty disc compression, uses laser energy to remove disc tissue. Laser disc compression has up to an 80 percent success rate. Spinal fusion is a surgical procedure in which two vertebrae are joined together. It might be used for conditions such as spondylolisthesis. A laminectomy is an operation performed to relieve pressure on one or more nerve roots in the lower spine area. The X-STOP implant is designed to keep the space between the spinous processes open so that when spinal stenosis patients stand upright, the nerves of the lumbar spines will have enough room and will not be painful.

Nerve blocks and spinal cord stimulation

Nerve blocks and spinal cord stimulation, both described earlier in this chapter, are two of the most commonly used pain control systems that require surgery. Nerve blocks can be used for localized pain, pain for a broader area like the back or legs, or for complex regional pain syndrome. Spinal cord stimulation patients normally experience a 50-70 percent reduction in pain. Neither procedure is a cure for chronic pain, but they can be used on a temporary basis without the long-term limitations of more invasive surgery, such as increased pain and reduced mobility.

Intradiscal electrothermal therapy (IDET)

Intradiscal electrothermal therapy (IDET) is a procedure used at Cleveland Clinic that ablates small nerve endings in the intervertebral discs and prevents nerves from sending pain messages to the brain (see Box 3-11). A catheter with an attached heating element is passed through a needle to the painful disc. The heat shrinks the collagen fibers surrounding the disc and provides pain relief. IDET is an option for some patients who would normally be candidates for spinal fusion. Although IDET is much less invasive

BOX 3-11: INTRADISCAL ELECTROTHERMAL THERAPY

Intradiscal electrothermal therapy (IDET) is used in patients with painful degenerative discs to remove the pain sensors in the disc and prevent nerves from sending pain messages to the brain.

BOX 3-12: TRANSDISCAL BIACUPLASTY

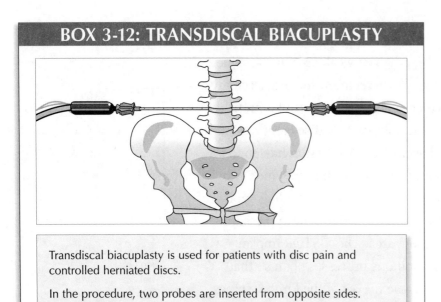

Transdiscal biacuplasty is used for patients with disc pain and controlled herniated discs.

In the procedure, two probes are inserted from opposite sides.

BOX 3-13: VERTEBROPLASTY

In 20 percent of patients with compression fractures in the spine that do not heal, vertebroplasty may be the only treatment option.

than most back surgeries, healing will still take several weeks. Pain relief is not immediate, and discomfort actually can increase for a day or two after the procedure. Gradually the pain from the procedure should diminish. IDET can be a useful, safe, and cost-effective option to treat chronic lower back pain.

Transdiscal biacuplasty

A related procedure, transdiscal biacuplasty is used for patients with disc pain and contained herniated discs (see Box 3-12). Two probes are inserted directly into the disc. Radiofrequency energy passes between the two probes and heats tissue. A built-in water-cooling system allows radiofrequency energy to heat a larger volume of disc tissue than with other methods. This new technique is promising to provide relief to millions of disabled patients.

Preliminary results are encouraging. A Cleveland Clinic study performed on 15 patients showed the procedure appeared to be an effective, minimally-invasive procedure for the treatment of disc pain in the back. Following treatment, more than half of the pilot study patients reduced the intensity of pain. They also improved their physical function by more than 50 percent.

Vertebroplasty and kyphoplasty

In vertebroplasty, a minimally-invasive surgical procedure done on an outpatient basis, medical-grade bone cement is injected into the spine to stabilize the fractured bone of a patient with osteoporosis (see Box 3-13). After the cement hardens, the crushed bone fragments fuse together, no longer rubbing against nerve endings. The procedure has a success rate of approximately 80 percent. One drawback is that vertebroplasty can increase the risk of additional fractures in adjacent vertebrae.

Kyphoplasty is a minimally-invasive technique for treating pain caused by compression fractures of the spine. A small tube and then an inflatable balloon are inserted into the vertebra (see Box 3-14). The balloon is inflated to re-establish some of the lost vertebral height, then the balloon is removed and the cavity that is created is filled with medical-grade cement. Kyphoplasty improves vertebral stability and often eliminates the need for braces and other forms of treatment. The procedure is followed by a period of rehabilitation and physical therapy, but most patients are encouraged to resume normal activities as soon as possible. Older adults with osteoporosis-related spinal fractures who had kyphoplasty have reported improvements in pain, daily functioning, and quality of life.

Radiofrequency ablation

Radiofrequency ablation (RFA) is a procedure in which pain is reduced by a radio-wave-generated, continuous electrical current that heats an area of nerve tissue and blocks pain signals originating from that spot. Ablation has been successful in treating chronic lower back pain, neck pain, and joint pain caused by arthritis. RFA is successful 70 percent of the time, and the effects can last from six months to several years. Although there is a slight risk of infection and bleeding at the site of insertion, most patients tolerate the procedure well and are not likely to have complications.

Pulsed radiofrequency (PRF) is a variation of RFA that uses short bursts of electrical current instead of a continuous flow. PRF may be an option for patients with intractable hip pain. PRF yields 'significant improvements' for patients with a herniated disc and spinal stenosis. Cooled radiofrequency is the most recent advance in neuroablation technology. It provides adequate therapeutic effects and also ensures less chance of neural damage. It has been effective to treat problems related to sacroiliac joint arthritis. The technique is currently being developed to treat pain secondary to thoracic facet arthritis.

Radiosurgery

Stereotactic radiosurgery delivers a highly concentrated dose of ionizing radiation to the root of the nerve. It is noninvasive and can avoid many of the risks and complications of open surgery and other treatments. Over time, the radiation exposure causes a lesion to develop in the nerve, which interrupts the transmission of pain signals to the brain. Radiosurgery appears to offer an effective treatment option for patients with trigeminal neuralgia.

BOX 3-14: KYPHOPLASTY

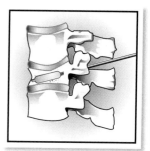

In kyphoplasty, a small tube with a balloon is inserted into the vertebra.

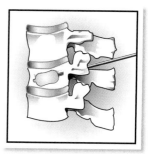

The balloon is inflated to create more space then removed.

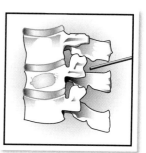

A medical grade cement is then injected to fill the space.

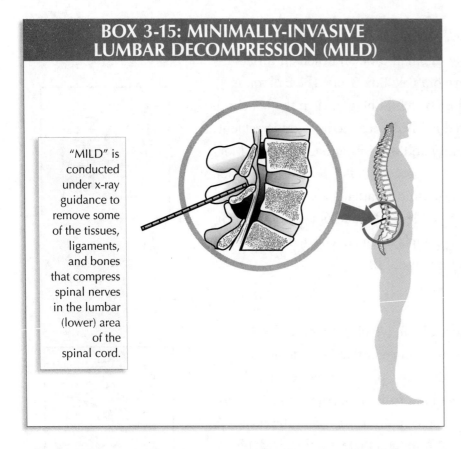
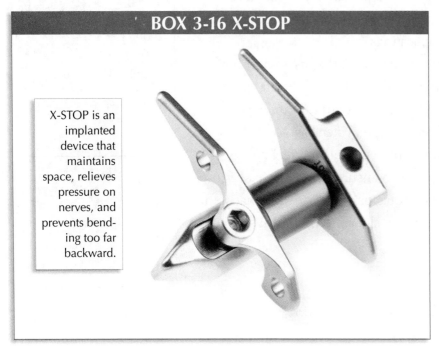
Mininally-invasive lumbar decompression (MILD)

Minimally-invasive lumbar decompression (MILD) is conducted through the guidance of fluoroscopic technology to remove some of the tissue and bone material that are compromising the size of the lumbar spinal canal in and around the spinal cord in the lumbar (lower back) area. Patients who are candidates for MILD are usually older adults (see Box 3-15).

Interspinous process decompression system (X-STOP)

In X-STOP, a titanium implant is inserted into an area of the spinal cord that has narrowed and put pressure on nerve roots. The device prevents patients from bending too far backward, which is a position that can cause leg pain, lower back pain, or both. The implant still allows flexion (bending forward) and limited rotation. X-STOP may be an option to open back surgery (see Box 3-16).

The MILD procedure has a definite advantage over the X-STOP, which is the lack of inserting hardware between the spines of the lumbar area. ∎

4 COMPLEMENTARY AND ALTERNATIVE PAIN MANAGEMENT

Approximately 40 percent of Americans use some form of complementary or alternative medicine (CAM), according to the National Institutes of Health and the Centers for Disease Control and Prevention. When prayer for a person's health is included in the definition of CAM, the number increases to 62 percent.

CAM refers to health systems, practices, and products that are not considered to be part of conventional medicine. The Cleveland Clinic and other medical institutions now include healthcare professionals who were once considered to be practitioners of alternative medicine.

The National Center for Complementary and Alternative Medicine makes a distinction between complementary and alternative medicine. Complementary medicine is used together with conventional medicine, whereas alternative medicine is used in place of conventional medicine.

This chapter discusses acupuncture, acupressure, biofeedback, chiropractic, copper bracelets, dimethyl sulfoxide (DMSO), glucosamine and chondroitin, hypnosis, magnets, massage, meditation, music, tai chi, and yoga.

Acupuncture

Many American doctors now include acupuncture in their practices, and others are learning how to do it or referring patients to licensed practitioners. Studies have shown it to have various degrees of effectiveness in treating fibromyalgia, knee osteoarthritis, tension and migraine headaches, lower back pain, and myofascial pain. *The Cochrane Library* has reported that acupuncture can provide patients who suffer from tension and migraine headaches some relief for their pain.

The journal *Brain Research* (February 5, 2010) reported that acupuncture has a significant effect on specific neural structures in the brain. Researchers in Great Britain determined that acupuncture deactivates areas in the brain that process pain, and that this could lead to a better understanding of how acupuncture works (see Box 4-1).

Not everyone responds to acupuncture therapy, just as everyone does not respond well to other types of treatments. For example, a recent review of studies published in the journal *Rheumatology* did not find sufficient evidence to recommend the procedure as a treatment for fibromyalgia, although the

---

NEW FINDING

Box 4-1: Acupuncture deactivates area of brain associated with pain

Acupuncture has a significant effect on specific neural structures in the brain, according to a report in the journal *Brain Research*. Researchers at the University of York and Hull York Medical School found that when a patient receives acupuncture treatment, a sensation called deqi occurs. This action deactivates parts of the brain that play a role in processing pain messages. The researchers say that the findings provide scientific evidence that acupuncture has specific effects within the brain. (*Brain Research*, February 5, 2010)

Box 4-2: Not enough evidence to support acupuncture for treatment of fibromyalgia

Although acupuncture may help some people who suffer from fibromyalgia, the evidence is not strong enough to recommend the procedure as a treatment for all, according to researchers in Germany who reviewed seven studies and the medical records of 385 subjects. The investigators also concluded that, at this time, acupuncture has not been shown to help with sleep disorders, fatigue, or physical functions of daily life. One reason for not recommending acupuncture is that in one of the studies, sham and simulated acupuncture resulted in better outcomes than real acupuncture. The authors do not rule out the possibility that acupuncture is effective for some people and some conditions, but say that more studies are needed before recommending it to the general population. (*Rheumatology*, January 25, 2010)

BOX 4-3: ACUPUNCTURE MERIDIANS

Acupuncture is based on the premise that a system of energy travels through channels, or meridians, in the body. Stimulating pressure points along those meridians can help heal the body.

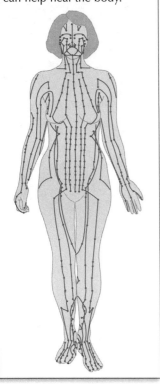

authors did not rule out the possibility that it may work for some people (see Box 4-2).

Acupuncture is not recommended for people who are taking certain drugs or who are extremely anxious. It also is not appropriate for conditions such as head injuries, herniated discs, or unstable joints.

Acupuncture treats illness or provides local anesthesia by inserting needles for 10 to 30 minutes at specific sites on channels, or meridians, that correspond with internal organs (see Box 4-3). The effect, in theory, is to create a 'life force' or energy balance to influence the progress of a disease or a condition such as chronic pain.

Electroacupuncture delivers an electrical current through acupuncture needles to restore the flow of energy throughout the body. Research conducted at the Yale School of Medicine determined that 30 minutes is the optimum time for electroacupuncture effectiveness (see Box 4-4).

Acupuncture treatment ranges from relatively painless to uncomfortable. The needles are half the thickness of those used to give injections and produce a sensation more like an insect bite than a shot. Adverse side effects are rare, but may include bleeding, infection, and dizziness.

If you decide to seek treatment, ask your physician to recommend a licensed acupuncturist who is certified by the American Academy of Medical Acupuncture (AAMA).

Acupressure

Acupressure is based on the same premise as acupuncture, except that stimulation is provided by touch rather than needles. When pressure is applied at specific points on the body, it can (in theory) rebalance the body's energy flow. Shiatsu is a Japanese form of acupressure.

A limited amount of evidence supports the practice of acupressure for pain control, relaxation, and stress management. One study showed that people with chronic low-back pain who were treated with acupressure had an 89 percent greater reduction in disability compared to those in a physical therapy group. Two other studies have shown limited success in using the practice to treat pain.

A Mayo Clinic researcher concluded that acupuncture and myofascial trigger point therapy treat essentially the same areas of the body.

Trigger point therapy involves pressure placed on tender muscle or trigger point regions.

Biofeedback

Biofeedback measures body functions such as breathing and heart rate, which are related to emotional stress and chronic pain. Becoming aware of the physical changes that take place when you are under stress or feel pain can help you to manage those variables.

Electrodes placed on the body measure your breathing rate, heart rate, blood pressure, skin temperature, and muscle tension. A monitor displays the results for you and the person administering the process. He or she will show you which body function levels indicate abnormalities, and will then teach you how to lower those indicators using techniques such as controlled breathing, imagery, and exercises. The idea is for you to gain control over these body functions and, in the process, self-treat a variety of physical problems, including chronic pain.

Biofeedback is not effective for certain kinds of pain, including acute lower-back pain, and not enough evidence exists to suggest that the technique is any more or less effective than any other pain management method. However, supplemental therapy that teaches coping and biofeedback skills can reduce pain, the potential for pain, and healthcare costs.

Federal health officials classify biofeedback as 'investigational'—not a medical necessity—but the technique can be useful when combined with medication and relaxation therapies.

Chiropractic

More than 50 percent of health maintenance organizations, more than 75 percent of private health plans, and all state workers' compensation systems cover chiropractic treatment. Chiropractors can bill Medicare, and about half the states cover chiropractic treatment under Medicaid. Forty percent of American patients seek chiropractic treatment for lower back pain.

Chiropractic care focuses on the relationship between the body's structure, particularly the spine, and function. Typically, chiropractors use a manual form of therapy called manipulation (or adjustment) to treat back pain, neck pain, headaches, sports injuries, and repetitive-use injuries. Back pain seems to get the most attention. The goal of most chiropractic care is to restore lost range of motion in a joint of the back. The idea is to make a 'motion segment' (two vertebrae and the disc that separates them) more flexible, rather than trying to return the spine to an ideal position.

Research on chiropractic treatment for lower back pain suggests that chiropractic adjustments can relieve acute pain as effectively as over-the-counter pain relievers or physical therapy, but they aren't effective for chronic pain. Also, people who are most likely to benefit from manipulation experience pain symptoms for approximately two weeks or less. A study conducted in Australia and published in the April, 2010 issue of *The Cochrane Library* says that spinal manipulation combined with other therapies relieves lower back pain, but the study did not identify which, if any, of the multiple approaches is most effective (see Box 4-5).

The risk of complications from adjustments of the lower back is very low, but the danger appears to be higher for adjustments of the neck. One study in the journal *Spine* found that patients who received chiropractic manipulation in the neck area experienced more adverse symptoms, such as increased neck pain, stiffness, headache, and radiating pain than people who received the gentler, massage-like spinal mobilization technique.

Similarities and differences exist between medical doctors (MDs) and chiropractors (DCs). Both take medical histories, conduct physical examinations, use similar diagnostic procedures, and recommend strengthening and stretching exercises. The medical doctor can prescribe medicine and perform surgery. The chiropractor can't. The physician addresses problems from a disease perspective and attempts to find a cure. The chiropractor tries to improve the function of daily activities, increase flexibility, and reduce pain, rather than cure a disease. The chiropractor believes that function can be restored in many cases by manipulating the spine, thus assisting the body in healing itself. The physician normally doesn't accept that theory. Increasingly, however, medical doctors and chiropractors are working together on the same pain management team.

Consider these factors before deciding whether or not you need chiropractic care for chronic pain:

■ **Trust.** If you think chiropractors can help, they probably will. If not, your chances for pain relief are not as good.

■ **Nature of your condition.** A number of conditions, including fractures, infections, and tumors, should only be treated by medical doctors.

■ **Risk level.** If your bones have become weakened due to advanced age or osteoporosis, chiropractic treatment may not be appropriate.

■ **Scope of practice.** You're better off with a chiropractor who treats musculoskeletal problems. Also look for someone who stresses good alignment through posture, ergonomics, stretching, and exercising.

Copper bracelets

Copper bracelets are enormously popular among those who believe that they relieve pain, but no evidence exists to support their effectiveness. Manufacturers claim, without any scientific basis, that tiny amounts of copper move through the surface of the skin and neutralize molecules that can damage cells in and around joints.

A study in the October, 2009 issue of *Complementary Therapies in Medicine* found no difference in the effect on pain, stiffness, or the need for medication when using a magnetic wrist strap, a weak magnetic wrist strap, a placebo strap, or a copper bracelet. A group of 45 subjects over the age of 50 tried the devices for 16 weeks.

Copper bracelets are not harmful and they may have a placebo effect, but until legitimate studies prove otherwise, they have no medical value. As one Cleveland Clinic physician said, "There is no risk except to your pocketbook and there is a 50 percent chance copper bracelets and magnets will make your pain better (because of the placebo effect)."

DMSO (dimethyl sulfoxide)

DMSO is an industrial solvent that can rapidly penetrate the skin and enhance the absorption of other substances, such as analgesics and steroids. Veterinarians use it on animals, but some people also use DMSO topically to treat muscle soreness. It enters the circulatory system quickly, causing an increased flow of blood to the affected area. Users report a garlic taste within seconds of its application. The practice is dangerous because it is impossible to know what other substances might be included in the solvent, and because DMSO is strong enough to cause severe skin burns. It is also toxic when taken internally. Studies of DMSO for pain relief are inconclusive, and doctors do not recommend its use.

Glucosamine and chondroitin

The National Institutes of Health study titled the Glucosamine/Chondroitin Intervention Trial (GAIT) provided mixed results regarding the benefits of glucosamine and chondroitin. Five years later, we are no closer to conclusive evidence on either substance. Both are found in and around the cells of cartilage that may help in its repair and maintenance. Glucosamine might also inhibit inflammation and stimulate cartilage cell resilience. GAIT found that the two supplements did little to alleviate mild knee osteoarthritis (OA) pain. However, a sub-group of the 1,600 subjects who had moderate-to-severe pain reported that the substances did help.

A series of studies published since the GAIT report have shown promising, but not conclusive evidence regarding the effectiveness of glucosamine and chondroitin for arthritis pain. Here are the highlights:

- *Annals of Internal Medicine* found no evidence that chondroitin alone prevents or reduces joint pain, but it did not rule out the possibility that it might be effective in patients with less severe arthritis pain.
- *American Family Physician* suggested that both glucosamine and chondroitin may improve symptoms of osteoarthritis, but there was no reliable evidence that taking the two substances together is more effective than taking them separately.
- *Annals of Internal Medicine* reported that glucosamine had little effect on arthritis of the hip.
- *Arthritis & Rheumatism* found that long-term use of prescription level doses of chondroitin reduced knee pain and slowed the process of joint narrowing.

For those who choose to take glucosamine and chondroitin supplements, the most commonly recommended dosages are 1,500 mg of glucosamine and 1,200 mg of chondroitin daily. The two substances are often combined in one pill.

The general consensus regarding glucosamine and chondroitin is that they may not be effective for mild knee OA, but they may be effective in reducing moderate-to-severe knee OA, and they don't have any apparent negative side effects. It takes 30-90 days to determine whether one or both of these substances will help relieve your pain.

Any information available on glucosamine and chondroitin at this point should be considered incomplete and inconclusive. The NIH and other institutions continue to research the effects of these substances on pain.

Hypnotherapy/hypnosis

Proponents of hypnotherapy stress that this method of pain management is not the kind of entertainment version of hypnosis seen on television or in a stage show. The patient does not look at an object in motion, act or speak in an embarrassing manner, lose consciousness, or follow directions against his or her will.

Hypnosis is a form of heightened concentration in which the patient is unusually receptive to behavior-changing suggestions, either from the therapist or from something the patient has written or recorded for later use. It is also described as a 'refined form of applied imagination.' The goal is to solve a problem, which in this case is to manage pain.

Hypnosis can be directed by a therapist or practiced by the patient acting alone. It can be taught by a professional or learned by studying self-hypnosis in a book.

There is evidence that self-hypnosis activates certain parts of the brain. Some think hypnosis may be able to change people's expectations about the degree of pain, altering the whole pain experience thereafter. Others believe that, by allowing a person to focus on an image, hypnosis blocks the perception of pain. Everyone agrees that hypnosis puts the person into a deep state of relaxation.

The NIH and the American Psychology Association have endorsed hypnosis as an alternative treatment for pain. A summary of studies, including one in *The Lancet*, showed that most patients feel pain relief after receiving hypnotic suggestions. Other studies have indicated that hypnosis is effective for relieving pain caused by cancer, irritable bowel syndrome, and surgery. *Psychology Health* has reported that hypnosis, biofeedback, relaxation therapy, and counseling all play roles in improving psychological outcomes and reducing pain.

Some people do not seem to be responsive to hypnosis. One study found that people who suffer from neuropathic (nerve) damage are more likely to benefit from it than others. In addition, there is no national certification of hypnotherapists, and finding a psychologist or other health professional qualified to practice hypnotherapy can be difficult.

Magnets

Magnet manufacturers claim their products are effective in treating fibromyalgia, back pain, headaches, neck pain, knee pain, and foot pain, but the scientific evidence to prove these claims does not exist. The National Center for Complementary and Alternative Medicine says, "There is no convincing scientific evidence to support claims that magnets can relieve pain of any type."

Studies of magnet use in very specific populations (polio patients, people with degenerative knee pain, women with low-back pain, and diabetic patients) have shown the treatment to be therapeutic. However, other studies have shown no benefit. It may be that any positive results seen in studies are a result of the placebo effect. Any treatment is more likely to work if people believe that it will.

There is no research to specify how strong the magnets should be, how long they should be applied, whether they could be harmful, or exactly how they work. Some researchers think magnets expand the size of blood vessels and increase blood flow. Others theorize that magnets create an electromagnetic field that helps relieve pain and speed up healing. Experts do agree that using magnets within six inches of a pacemaker is very dangerous. Low-intensity 'therapeutic magnets' placed a safe distance from pacemakers, however, appear to do no harm.

Magnetic stimulation, as opposed to simply wearing magnets or taping them to certain parts of the body, may have promise for reducing pain. At Albert Einstein College of Medicine, a group of scientists found that a hand-held device that delivers a magnetic impulse to the back of the head significantly reduced migraine headache pain (see Box 4-6).

Massage

The connection between massage and pain relief is not clear, but the practice may have some therapeutic value. Previous research has shown that:

- Massage therapy was effective in reducing the frequency of tension headaches, but not in easing the intensity of those headaches.
- Fibromyalgia patients who had a massage three times a week for five weeks experienced significantly less pain, anxiety, and depression than a control group.
- Massage reduced pain better than acupuncture and relaxation exercises.
- Massage appears to ease lower back pain, osteoarthritis, and fibromyalgia, as well as other conditions such as cancer-related pain, post-surgical pain, and headaches.
- Massage can, in the short term, reduce pain, increase circulation, reduce muscle tension, and improve range of motion. However, massage cannot cure or reverse the course of any disease.

If you decide to try therapeutic massage, talk with your doctor first, check to see that your therapist is qualified, and make sure that massage will not compromise other treatments you are receiving. Finally, go into massage therapy with a positive attitude and with realistic expectations about what massage can and cannot do for you.

Meditation

As is the case with many treatments for chronic pain, no one knows how meditation works. It cannot take pain away, but various studies have indicated that meditation can reduce stress, relax muscles, slow breathing, reduce episodes of depression, enhance immune response, and diminish awareness of pain. Nevertheless, few studies have been conclusive, and further research is needed to show any real benefit. One new study at the University of North Carolina (*Journal of Pain*, March 15, 2010) found that training in meditation practices for three days produced relaxed states and reduced pain when a group of subjects were exposed to painful stimuli (see Box 4-7).

Two commonly used methods of meditation involve concentration techniques and 'mindfulness.' In the concentration model, you silently or quietly repeat a word, sound, or thought to help you focus. Extraneous thoughts or feelings (like pain) are not allowed in. When your attention wanders, you return your mind to its original object of concentration. In mindfulness meditation, you focus on a single thought or process (like breathing) and slowly expand your awareness to include thoughts, feelings, and body sensations (other than pain). Mindfulness meditation is used for stress reduction at more than 250 hospitals and clinics in the U.S.

Meditation, although seemingly simple, takes discipline and daily practice to shut out the distractions of the outside world. This difficulty is reflected in the relatively few people who practice it. Although meditation is classified here as an alternative form of therapy, respected institutions like Harvard, Stanford, and Cleveland Clinic have acknowledged its value when used by the right patients. Meditation and related activities in some people can produce a relaxation response and physiological changes that could reverse the effects of stress, including pain.

NEW FINDING

Box 4-7: Meditation may bring pain relief

Researchers at the University of North Carolina found that creating a relaxed state of mind can enhance the body's ability to deal with pain. Subjects were trained in meditation techniques for three days and then exposed (voluntarily) to painful stimuli. Relaxed states produced by brief periods of mindfulness meditation sessions reduced pain ratings. The participants had less reaction to both low and high pain intensities and showed significant reductions in anxiety levels after each meditation session. (*Journal of Pain*, March 15, 2010)

Music

Research conducted at Cleveland Clinic has shown that listening to music can have a significant effect on chronic pain and depression. It can also make people feel more in control of their pain and less disabled by their condition. Specifically, experimental groups that incorporated music into their pain management strategy reported that their pain fell by between 12 and 21 percent. Depression occurred 19 to 25 percent less in music groups than in control groups that did not use music as complementary pain therapy.

Prolotherapy

There are several types of prolotherapy, but to treat chronic pain it is a procedure in which a substance, frequently dextrose- or saline-based, is injected into an area of the body in an effort to stimulate the body to start its own healing process. It has been used for knee, shoulder, and lower back pain, among others.

As with almost every alternative or complementary treatment, the evidence regarding the success of prolotherapy is mixed. Prolotherapy injections have been found to be no more effective than a placebo in controlling lower back pain. Prolotherapy combined with spinal manipulation, exercise, and other therapies has resulted in better results for lower back pain compared to control groups, and prolotherapy for chronic shoulder pain caused by tendinitis, according to some studies, is very effective.

Tai chi

Tai chi combines relaxation, meditation, and deep breathing with slow, gentle, continuous, and very structured exercises called forms. 'Standing, graceful postures,' 'achieving harmony between body and mind,' and 'meditation in motion' are some of the phrases used to describe tai chi movements.

The art can help improve balance, overcome a fear of falling, reduce blood pressure, and provide a general sense of well-being. It is especially effective in older adults, because they can practice tai chi at different intensity levels.

Increasingly, tai chi has become a form of exercise recommended for those with chronic pain, but direct evidence that it reduces pain is sketchy. Indirectly, exercise of any kind seems to reduce pain, so tai chi qualifies in that respect. There is some evidence that tai chi reduces the amount of stress hormones the body produces and general anecdotal evidence that it reduces stress. Researchers are investigating possible benefits for the immune system, respiratory system, arthritis, sleep, and bone loss. A Westernized form of tai chi may boost immunity against shingles and reduced the pain of the disease. Tai chi may relieve pain among people who suffer from severe knee osteoarthritis.

The number of movements in tai chi varies from 18 to more than 100. You can start learning with a five-minute session once a week and work up to the target goal. Finding a qualified instructor is a challenge because there is no standard certification for teachers. Too many people who are 'teaching' tai chi have taken only a one-weekend workshop.

To enroll in a class, call a YMCA/YWCA, health facility, college or university, or city recreation department. Don't sign up for sessions until you are certain that tai chi is a good fit for you. If possible, observe a class or take a trial class.

For most people, tai chi appears to be a safe, body-friendly activity. However, anyone who has acute chest pain with minimal exertion, severe shortness of breath, dizziness or fainting spells, or uncontrolled blood pressure, should seek the advice of a physician before starting tai chi, as should people who have osteoporosis, acute back pain, or active infections.

Yoga

Yoga uses movement, meditation, relaxation, and gentle breathing, all of which contribute to one's sense of self-awareness. The American Pain Foundation calls it 'an ancient method of stilling the mind.' For some, yoga is more of a spiritual experience; for others, it's an alternative exercise that promotes flexibility, strength, and endurance. In one principle of yoga, called 'contraction and release,' certain postures are held, then released. In doing so, according to yoga proponents, physical and emotional barriers dissolve, allowing energy to move to areas of chronic pain. The percentage of Americans who have used yoga continues to increase.

At Arizona State University, yoga-type slow breathing techniques reduced pain intensity in groups of healthy women and among women with fibromyalgia. The research was published in the April 2010 issue of the journal *PAIN* (see Box 4-8).

Yoga is often studied in combination with other alternative interventions, making it difficult to isolate the practice as the single reason for improvement. Under certain conditions, yoga has been shown to relieve pain caused by carpal tunnel syndrome, headaches, fibromyalgia, and osteoarthritis of the hands. *The Journal of Family Practice* found that 69 percent of patients who performed yoga experienced an improvement in back pain symptoms. The journal *Headache* found that yoga, in combination with breathing techniques, relaxation exercises, and meditation, reduced the frequency and intensity of migraine headaches. A case can be made for the indirect effects of yoga on chronic pain. Because many of those who suffer from chronic pain also experience depression, yoga could have some value in addressing both conditions. An important component of yoga is breathing technique. Specific breathing exercises are thought to serve as mood elevators, as well as tools to calm the central nervous system. Some people use yoga to escape depression, or to calm their nerves and thereby ease their chronic pain.

Yoga, like tai chi, Pilates, and other forms of traditional or alternative exercise, has a role to play in the treatment of chronic pain for some people. For it to be effective, you have to make sure the technique is a good match for your personality and physical condition. Yoga requires time, training, and practice. Depending on the cause of your chronic pain, you may have to ask the instructor to help you modify or avoid certain positions in order to prevent undue stress on joints and muscles. ∎

NEW FINDING

Box 4-8: Slow breathing techniques may reduce moderate pain

Researchers at Arizona State University found that yoga-style slow breathing and meditation may help control chronic pain. The study is believed to be the first to directly examine the benefits of breathing rate on physical and emotional pain. Two groups of women were subjected to brief pulses of moderately painful heat on their palms. Twenty-seven participants were fibromyalgia patients; 25 were not. Slow breathing reduced ratings of pain intensity in most of the subjects, as well as negative emotion, in both groups, but the greatest effect was among those who did not have fibromyalgia. Only those who reported having consistent positive emotion in their lives felt less pain while breathing at half their normal rates. The authors believe that learning breathing techniques may have applications for not only fibromyalgia, but for other types of pain such as osteoarthritis and lower back pain. *(PAIN, April, 2010)*

5 EXERCISE, DIET, AND WEIGHT CONTROL OPTIONS

Exercise, diet, and weight control are proven, cost-effective methods of managing chronic pain. Exercise in particular is a great way to address chronic pain and share in healthy social experiences. New studies described in this chapter show how exercise and nutrition can have a specific effect on conditions such as arthritis, fibromyalgia, and lower back pain.

Exercise

Exercise stimulates the body to release powerful endorphins that keep pain signals from reaching the brain. Additional benefits include weight control, increased energy levels, better sleep patterns, and less anxiety and depression. All of these factors are directly or indirectly related to chronic pain management, regardless of a person's age.

Six months of aerobic exercise and weightlifting can result in an increase in aerobic fitness and strength. Resistance training can have a positive impact on the perception of pain, and it can significantly increase strength, flexibility, and agility in adults who are well into their eighties. Women over 70 could reduce the incidence of arthritis pain by staying physically active. Even a modest exercise program can lower heart rate, reduce anxiety, and improve mood in chronic pain patients. Unfortunately, exercise is commonly underused as a treatment for chronic pain, especially in cases involving the back and neck. Conversely, two research teams in Maryland and Michigan showed that 30 minutes of physical activity five days a week resulted in improved physical function and less pain. The findings appeared in *Arthritis Research & Therapy*, March 30, 2010 (see Box 5-1).

NEW FINDING

Box 5-1: Physical activity improves physical function and reduces pain in adults with fibromyalgia

In a 12-week trial that involved 84 participants, those who accumulated 30 minutes of self-selected physical activity five days a week reported significant and clinically relevant changes in physical function and pain caused by fibromyalgia. Their results were compared to a control group that received only information and support. The study was conducted at Johns Hopkins University School of Medicine and at the University of Michigan Chronic Pain & Fatigue Research Center. The authors of the study also investigated the relationship between exercise and fatigue, body mass index, depression, tenderness, and a six-minute walk test. The only difference between the control and experimental groups were related to physical function and pain, although the subjects increased their average number of daily steps by 54 percent. (*Arthritis Research & Therapy*, March 30, 2010)

Exercise doesn't have to involve high-intensity physical exertion. Mild-to-moderate-intensity exercise performed at home or at a health center has a record of reducing chronic pain. There are three basic types of exercise and each should be in your program:

- **Resistance training** increases muscle strength and muscle endurance and may even reverse the aging process in muscle tissue. Strength training can reduce chronic neck pain.
- **Flexibility exercises** are especially helpful to people with arthritis-related pain.
- **Endurance (aerobic) exercise** includes any kind of physical activity that causes the heart to beat faster than normal (within a safe range) for extended periods of time.

Resistance training

Resistance training includes lifting weights, performing modified push-ups, sit-ups, or other body weight exercises using elastic bands, or any other type of equipment that provides resistance.

The combination of resistance training and water exercises might provide additional benefits. The water helps to support the body and takes pressure off weight-bearing joints. Exercising in a heated swimming pool could be an option for treating fibromyalgia. Stretching and exercises in warm water relieved pain and daily function in people with knee or hip osteoarthritis. A new study in the April 10, 2010, issue of the *Journal of the American College of Sports Medicine* showed that exercises specifically designed for lower back muscles—not other muscle groups—could be a solution to some cases of lower back pain (see Box 5-2).

NEW FINDING

Box 5-2: Exercises specifically designed for lower back muscles may relieve chronic back pain

Floor exercises and an exercise machine designed specifically to strengthen back muscles (and not other muscle groups) may provide a partial remedy for lower back pain. Researchers at the University of Montreal instructed subjects between the ages of 18 and 65 to complete various exercises and then used electromyography sensors to measure the level of activity and fatigue in certain muscles. They were able to target fatigued muscles, even though those muscles were not yet showing a decrease in strength. Types of exercises included those performed on a machine designed to strengthen back muscles while in a semi-sitting position and one that used a cushion to stabilize the pelvis. (*Journal of the American College of Sports Medicine,* April 10, 2010)

BOX 5-3: CURLS

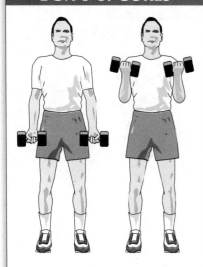

Hold a dumbbell in each hand, arms down, palms in, and feet comfortably apart. Bring the weights upward by bending your elbows and rotating your wrists outward. Slowly lower the weights and repeat the movement. Don't hold your breath while performing curls or any other exercise.

BOX 5-4: WALL SQUATS

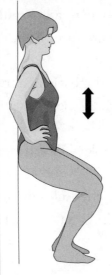

Stand close enough to a wall to lean back against it. Using the wall to support your back, slowly and slightly bend your knees and assume a modified squat position (not to the point at which your upper legs are parallel to the floor). Keep your heels apart, toes pointing slightly out, knees above your big toes, and hands resting on your hips. Do not try this exercise if you have a knee injury or condition that could be aggravated by a knee bend position.

BOX 5-5: SHRUGS

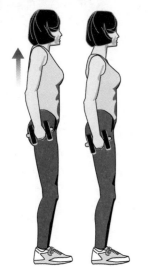

Grasp a dumbbell in each hand, arms down, palms in, feet comfortably spread. Shrug your shoulders up and as high as possible. Slowly return to the starting position and repeat. Perform eight lifts at first (if you can without pain) and gradually increase the number of repetitions.

BOX 5-6: HEEL RAISES

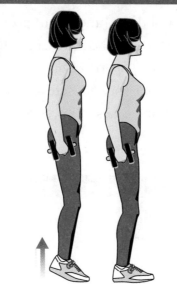

Hold a 3- to 8-pound dumbbell in each hand, arms down, palms in. Stand with your toes on a secure surface. Rise slowly on your toes while keeping your body erect and knees straight. Return to the starting position and repeat the movement.

It is not too late to begin a program of resistance training. Get your doctor's permission first, read the guidelines below, and choose the best exercises for your situation. You are more likely to stick with the program if you can find an exercise group made up of friends and acquaintances in your age group.

- **Equipment:** Very light dumbbells (held with one hand) or barbells (held with two hands) or weight machines, if you have access to a health facility
- **Resistance or amount of weight:** A weight you can lift 8-12 times with good form
- **Repetitions:** 8-12 repetitions
- **Sets (lifts before resting):** 1 at the beginning; 2-3 later
- **Frequency:** 2-3 times a week, but not on consecutive days
- **Increasing resistance:** Add 2.5 pounds when you can perform 12 repetitions in 2 consecutive sets with good form
- **Types of exercises:** Examples are curls and shrugs for the upper body, partial (wall) squats (with or without weights) for the trunk, and heel raises for the legs (see Boxes 5-3, 5-4, 5-5, 5-6).

Flexibility

Stretching programs should be individual in nature, depending on your level of fitness, existing flexibility, overall health, lifestyle, age, and degree of pain. Get your doctor's permission, read the guidelines below, and decide on the best stretches for you.

- **Time of day:** Generally, morning is best, but add sessions as needed and as your schedule allows
- **Frequency:** Daily, but don't worry if you occasionally miss a session or two
- **Intensity:** Stretch until you feel tension or resistance, then hold the stretch before returning to the starting position
- **Amount of time:** 30 seconds per stretch or 3 10-second stretches
- **Repetitions:** 2-3 repetitions
- **Types of stretches:** Examples are lunges for the trunk and lower body, sitting knees-to-chest for the trunk, sitting or standing twist for the trunk or upper body, and overhead reach for arms and shoulders (see Boxes 5-7, 5-8, 5-9, 5-10).

Aerobic exercise

Aerobic, or endurance, exercise may be the most important kind. Strength training and range-of-motion exercises are helpful, but neither does much for the cardiovascular system. By walking, swimming, cycling, or participating in other aerobic activities, you'll improve your strength, flexibility, and aerobic capacity. People who swim, walk, or bike at least three hours a week can reduce their lower back pain more efficiently than those who rely on specific back exercises.

To qualify as moderate-intensity exercise, your routine has to elevate your heart rate into a target zone and keep

BOX 5-10: KNEES TO CHEST

Lay on your back, pull your knees toward your chest, and hold for 20-30 seconds. Before you repeat the stretch, slowly move one leg at a time back to an extended position on the floor. A variation of this exercise is to assume the same position and bring one knee at a time toward your chest. You can also perform this stretch sitting in a chair and pulling one knee at a time up and toward your chest.

BOX 5-7: LUNGES

Stand with your feet separated by 12-18 inches, one foot in front of the other and toes pointed forward. Slowly shift your weight forward, bending the front knee and keeping the heel of the back foot on the floor. Switch leg positions and repeat. This stretch can also be a strength-training exercise by holding 3- to 8-pound dumbbells in each hand.

BOX 5-8: OVERHEAD REACH

Interlock your fingers. Lift your arms and rotate your wrists so the palms are facing the sky. Extend your arms as far upward as possible and hold for 20-30 seconds, then return to the starting position. You should feel a stretch in the upper part of your back and in the shoulders.

BOX 5-9: SITTING TWIST

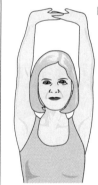

Sit erect in a straight chair. Cross your arms in front of your chest and rotate your shoulders as far to the left as you can without discomfort. Hold, return to the starting position, and repeat once or twice. Then rotate to the right. As you get used to the stretch, gradually increase the degree of rotation.

BOX 5-11

Determining target heart rate

Target heart rate is a very general guide to determine an appropriate heart rate per minute during exercise. The idea is to reach a target rate or zone and keep it there for approximately 30 minutes several times a week in order to maintain or improve your cardiovascular health. To determine your target heart zone, the American Heart Association (AHA) says to first subtract your age from 220. That will establish your maximum heart rate (the rate you do not want to exceed for any length of time). Multiply that number by .50 to .75, depending on your fitness level (closer to .50 if you are just beginning an aerobic exercise program; closer to .75 if you are a well-conditioned, serious exerciser; low .60s if you are in the middle). Below are examples from the AHA.

AGE	TARGET ZONE
40	90-135 beats/minute
50	85-128 beats/minute
60	80-120 beats/minute
70	75-113 beats/minute

it there for at least 30 minutes. See Box 5-11 to determine your target heart zone. Brisk walking (3.5 mph) is one way to do it and using a pedometer to count steps may be just the motivation you need to start walking on a daily basis. Patients suffering from chronic peripheral artery pain may show significant improvement when they engage in a supervised walking program (see Box 5-12).

To manage or lose body weight, you'll have to exercise for 60-90 minutes on most days of the week. In the government's 2005 dietary guidelines, described in the following section, regular exercise is an important part of the program. Regardless of the exercise you choose, talk with your doctor first and gradually work toward longer distances, duration, and intensity. Never increase any exercise component by more than

BOX 5-12: SAMPLE WALKING PROGRAM

	Session A (15 min.)	Walk slowly 5 min.	Then walk briskly 5 min.	Then walk slowly 5 min.
WEEK 1:	Session B (15 min.)	Walk slowly 5 min.	Then walk briskly 5 min.	Then walk slowly 5 min.
	Session C (15 min.)	Walk slowly 5 min.	Then walk briskly 5 min.	Then walk slowly 5 min.
WEEK 2:	17 min. total	Walk slowly 5 min.	Then walk briskly 7 min.	Then walk slowly 5 min.
WEEK 3:	19 min. total	Walk slowly 5 min.	Then walk briskly 9 min.	Then walk slowly 5 min.
WEEK 4:	21 min. total	Walk slowly 5 min.	Then walk briskly 11 min.	Then walk slowly 5 min.
WEEK 5:	23 min. total	Walk slowly 5 min.	Then walk briskly 13 min.	Then walk slowly 5 min.
WEEK 6:	25 min. total	Walk slowly 5 min.	Then walk briskly 15 min.	Then walk slowly 5 min.
WEEK 7:	28 min. total	Walk slowly 5 min.	Then walk briskly 18 min.	Then walk slowly 5 min.
WEEK 8:	30 min. total	Walk slowly 5 min.	Then walk briskly 20 min.	Then walk slowly 5 min.
WEEK 9:	33 min. total	Walk slowly 5 min.	Then walk briskly 23 min.	Then walk slowly 5 min.
WEEK 10:	36 min. total	Walk slowly 5 min.	Then walk briskly 26 min.	Then walk slowly 5 min.
WEEK 11:	38 min. total	Walk slowly 5 min.	Then walk briskly 28 min.	Then walk slowly 5 min.
WEEK 12+:	40 min. total	Walk slowly 5 min.	Then walk briskly 30 min.	Then walk slowly 5 min.

[from American Heart Association/NIH Publication No. 93-1677]

10 percent a week. Use this section as a guide to help you decide on the best aerobic exercise program for your needs.

- **Frequency:** At least 5 days a week
- **Intensity:** Hard enough to get your heart rate into its target zone
- **Amount of time:** 30–90 minutes a day (all at once or broken into smaller time segments)
- **Types of exercises:** Walking, swimming, water aerobics, cycling, and dancing

Diet and weight control

No single food or diet will reduce or eliminate chronic pain, but what you eat can affect a few painful conditions. Gout is related to high levels of uric acid, found in red meat and seafood. Consuming more dairy products decreases the risk of gout. Osteoporosis may be a result of calcium deficiencies. Women should get at least 1,500 mg of calcium daily; men 1,000 mg or more. Drinking milk, which contains the sleep-inducing substance tryptophan, might help fight insomnia, which is often a consequence of chronic pain. Opioid drugs used for chronic pain can cause constipation, which can be relieved by gradually increasing your intake of high-fiber foods (fruits, vegetables, cereals, brown rice).

Researchers at the Mayo Clinic found that inadequate vitamin D levels are associated with greater use of narcotic pain medications, which might indicate that chronic pain patients and their physicians should assess vitamin D status.

A well-balanced diet and exercise will help control your weight, which can have a dramatic effect on pain. People who are obese may be more sensitive to pain than those who are of normal weight. Even modest weight losses (15 pounds) in obese individuals can reduce the pain associated with knee osteoarthritis by almost 50 percent. A study published in the February 2010 edition of *Arthritis Care & Research* found that obesity and inactivity makes women more susceptible to osteoarthritis, and the May 2010 issue of the same journal reported that obesity increases the risk of fibromyalgia (see Boxes 5-13 and 5-14).

The Department of Health and Human Services and the Department of Agriculture have issued a report titled *Dietary Guidelines for Americans*. Here are the highlights:

- Consume a variety of 'nutrient-dense' foods (lean meat, fish, poultry, green vegetables, citrus fruits), while limiting the intake of saturated and trans fats, cholesterol, added sugars, salt, and alcohol.

- People over 50 should take vitamins D and B12 in fortified foods or supplements. Drink three cups per day of fat-free/low-fat milk, or substitute a nonfat or low-fat alternative, such as yogurt.

- Balance calories from foods and beverages with calories expended. Make small, systematic decreases in calories and progressive increases in physical activity. Although diet and exercise should go hand-in-hand, cutting calories alone can expedite weight loss. Eighty percent of the participants in a program titled EatRight were able to maintain their weight loss during two years of follow-up assessment.

- Older adults should participate in regular physical activity to reduce declines associated with aging. Engage in at least 30 minutes of moderate-intensity physical activity daily. To manage or lose body weight, exercise for 60-90 minutes on most days of the week.

- Eat two cups of fruit and two-and-a-half cups of vegetables daily. Eating low energy-dense foods such as fruits and vegetables can help you lose weight. Whole fruits are better than fruit juices because they contain more fiber. Choose dried beans, as well as dark-green (romaine lettuce, spinach), orange (carrots, sweet potatoes), and yellow (winter squash) vegetables.

- Get less than 10 percent of your total calories from saturated fatty acids and consume less than 300 mg per day of cholesterol. Keep trans fat consumption as low as possible. Total fat should not exceed 20 to 35 percent of calories, and most fats should come from healthy sources, such as fish, nuts, and vegetable oils.

- Eat at least three ounces of whole grain cereals, breads, pasta, and rice a day. Look for the words 'whole grain' high up, if not first, on the list of ingredients. Cut back on or skip white bread and rice.

- Consume less than 2,300 mg of sodium (about one teaspoon of salt) per day. Older Americans should limit salt intake to 1,500 mg.

- Eat enough fruits and vegetables so that you are getting 4,700 mg of potassium—the recommended dietary allowance.

- Drink alcohol in moderation or not at all.

Maintaining weight loss appears to be more effective and longer lasting when the person trying to lose weight has some sort of regular contact with a nutritionist or other healthcare provider. Even one brief telephone conversation a month can result in less 'regained' weight. ■

6 HOW TO GET HELP— WHAT TO EXPECT

Two out of ten people with chronic pain do not seek the help of a physician, and when the other eight people finally decide to get help, it's usually later rather than sooner. This may be one of the reasons why chronic pain is known for being under-treated. Whatever you do, don't fall into the 'I'll-know-when-it's-time' attitude. Few people know when the time to get treatment has come without the help of family members, friends, or healthcare professionals.

Here are some guidelines for knowing when it is time for a new approach to your pain problem:

- Routine tasks become difficult or impossible because of pain
- Your activities are increasingly limited because of pain
- You have recurring pain after a period of noticeable improvement
- You feel a loss of control over your pain
- You become angry, irritable, or frustrated because of your pain
- You feel guilty or lose self-esteem
- You limp, cry, groan, grimace, or talk about pain constantly

Several steps can speed up your decision to see a pain management specialist. One of the first is to ask your physician or surgeon if seeing a pain management specialist is appropriate. Make sure that the pain management specialist is board certified and fellowship trained in pain management. Your doctor is likely to refer you to a pain specialist. The majority of physicians are not trained in chronic pain care, and many are reluctant to treat it aggressively, particularly if the treatment involves potentially-addictive drugs.

Finding a pain management specialist

Ask your doctor to refer you to one or more pain management specialists. A pain management specialist is a medical doctor who specializes in the treatment of people who have ongoing pain. He or she could come from various specialties, often anesthesiology, but also neurology or rehabilitation medicine. Getting more than one name allows you to choose the doctor with whom you feel most comfortable because of age, gender, specialty, experience treating a friend or family member, or even location. If you are not comfortable with your physician's recommendation, ask a friend who has seen a pain management specialist about his or her experience and treatment results. Among those who treat pain exclusively are physiatrists (physical medicine and rehabilitation physicians), internists, anesthesiologists, neurologists, psychologists, psychiatrists, osteopaths, chiropractors, occupational therapists, and physical therapists.

Not every community has a standalone pain treatment center, clinic, or service. These facilities might instead be located in a wing of your local hospital or medical center, in a professional building, or in a doctor's office. The American Society of Anesthesiologists suggests that you try these sources for help locating a pain management specialist:

■ Call your local hospital and ask if it is affiliated with a pain treatment center.

■ If a pain management center is not available, ask your hospital to connect you to the Department of Anesthesiology.

■ If your hospital does not have information regarding a pain management center, contact the nearest school of medicine and ask if it has a pain research program.

■ On the Internet, contact the American Society of Anesthesiologists at www.asahq.org for information regarding pain centers nationwide.

Once you have decided on a specialist and made an appointment, you can prepare for the first visit. Make that visit more productive by creating a checklist (see Box 6-1). Get a copy of your medical records, as well as your lab test results, X-rays, MRIs, and other scans. Take pill containers or a list of every medication you are taking, including supplements and over-the-counter drugs. Take a friend or family member with you. A second person familiar with your condition might be able to provide information that you overlook, and can even help you get ready for the visit.

The first office visit

Before your first visit with a pain management specialist, do some mental homework. Honestly think about your situation. What do you think is wrong? What kind of help are you looking for? What is your goal? What do you think a new approach or a different doctor can offer?

The office visit to a pain management specialist will be similar to other first doctor visits. Arrive well ahead of the appointment time. You'll be asked to fill out several forms, so be sure to take a written reminder of previous illnesses, hospitalizations, surgery types and dates, medicines to which you are allergic, physical therapies, and contact information for you and your family members.

BOX 6-1

Checklist: 10 items to take to your pain management specialist visit

1. Photo ID

2. Medical records from previous doctors

3. List of prescription and over-the-counter medications you're taking

4. List of vitamins and supplements you're taking

5. Film from X-rays, CTs, MRIs, other scans

6. Lab test results

7. A list and dates of previous surgeries

8. List of questions to ask the doctor

9. Insurance card and/or Medicare card

10. Checkbook or credit card to pay for your visit

Make an actual list of questions you'd like to ask your doctor. Here are some examples provided by the American Chronic Pain Association:

- What do you believe is the cause of the pain?
- What might help relieve the pain?
- What are the pros and cons of each approach?
- What are possible side effects of treatments?
- What is the long-term outlook?
- What are my responsibilities?
- How should we communicate (office visits, telephone, e-mail)?
- Is there another person in your office who should be contacted?
- What part of my care will this person (physician or other) be responsible for—pain only or general medical care?
- Your pain management specialist will want you to describe your pain in as much detail as possible. Give some thought to explaining:
- The location of your pain (a drawing can be helpful and might be provided by the nurse or doctor)
- The type of pain (aching, throbbing, tingling, stabbing)
- The conditions (time of day, activity) that make the pain better or worse
- The duration of the pain (always present, worse at night or in the morning)
- The intensity of the pain (usually based on a 1-10 scale)

Measuring pain

There are three types of scales to help doctors diagnose and measure the intensity of pain. Visual scales either have pictures of the body to indicate where the pain is located, or drawings of facial expressions that correspond to the way one feels. The 'faces' scale—a range of happy-to-sad-faces—is especially useful for those who cannot use language to describe their pain.

Verbal pain scales allow the patient to use words such as mild, uncomfortable, moderate, intense, and severe to more precisely describe their pain. These scales are imprecise, however, because the same words can mean different things to different people.

Numerical scales require patients to assign a number to the intensity of pain they feel. The most common numerical scales range from 1-10, but others have numbers ranging from 1-5 or 1-6. Scales that include descriptive words and numbers are more effective than those that simply have 'no pain' on one end and 'worst possible pain' on the other. All pain scales involve some degree of subjectivity, so it is important that you and your doctor agree on the interpretation of pictures, words, or numbers.

Remember that these scales are snapshot measures. Describing how well you function on a day-to-day basis, your sleep patterns, and your use of analgesic medications are more accurate measures of the magnitude of your pain and the effectiveness of your treatment.

Pain Level	Description
0	No pain
1	Mild pain; you're aware of it, but it doesn't bother you
2	Moderate pain; tolerable without medications
3	Moderate pain; requires medication to tolerate
4-5	More severe pain; you begin to feel antisocial
6	Severe pain
7-9	Intensely severe pain
10	Most severe pain; unbearable

The exam

Expect the doctor to do more than the usual amount of pushing and probing to detect tender areas, and to put your body through various range-of-motion movements, especially if your pain seems to involve muscles and joints. You've probably seen it before, but don't be surprised if the doctor uses a rubber hammer to check the reflexes in your arms and legs. A neurological examination in the office might also involve testing your movement, reflexes, sensation, balance, and coordination. These shouldn't be uncomfortable.

Both you and your doctor should be aware of the possibility of referred pain. There are times when a problem with an internal organ can cause pain in an unlikely location. This happens because the painful area is served by nerves from the same part of the spinal cord as the organ. Knowledge of referred pain enables the physician to diagnose the real problem and take measures to correct it. Here are some examples:

Source of pain	Location of referred pain
Liver, gallbladder	Right shoulder blade, right side of neck, chest
Abdomen	Upper back, chest, right shoulder
Kidney	Back (below the ribs), groin
Heart	Neck, jaws, arms, shoulders, upper back
Feet	Lower legs, knees
Eyes	Head (headache)
Lower back	Hip, legs

Ears.................................Jaw (TMJ)
Heart................................Legs (in peripheral artery disease—PAD)
Knees...............................Hips, lower legs

Diagnostic tests

Although it would be nice if your doctor or other pain specialist could prescribe a treatment program based on one office visit, additional tests may be necessary. Among those tests are electrodiagnostic procedures that include electromyography (EMG), nerve conduction studies, and evoked potential (EP) studies. In EMG, thin needles are inserted into muscles and the doctor can see or listen to electrical signals displayed on an EMG machine. Information from EMG can help physicians tell precisely which muscles or nerves are affected by weakness or pain.

In nerve conduction tests, the doctor uses two sets of electrodes (similar to those used during an electrocardiogram). One set of electrodes is placed on the skin over the muscles. The second set is used to make a recording of the nerve's electrical signals, and from this information the doctor can determine whether there is nerve damage.

EP tests also involve two sets of electrodes—one set attached to a limb for stimulating a nerve, and another set on the scalp for recording the speed of nerve signal transmission to the brain.

Imaging, especially MRI, provides pictures of the body's structures and tissues. MRI uses magnetic fields and radio waves to differentiate between healthy and diseased tissue.

A thermography test measures the temperature of surface tissue as a function of blood flow. This test can be used to detect altered blood flow to a painful area, which may indicate a problem with the autonomic nervous system.

Finally, X-rays produce pictures of structures such as bones and joints. Discography and functional anesthetic discography (FAD) are included in this category (see Box 6-2). FAD is used to confirm the presence of damaged discs. When a patient moves in a way that causes pain, an anesthetic is injected in the disc to relieve the discomfort. If the pain is not alleviated, it either confirms the result of a discogram or indicates a false position finding.

Following all the tests and examinations, the pain management specialist will discuss treatment options with you. Those options can be as simple as trying a new medication or as complex as surgery. ▪

BOX 6-2

Diagnostic tests and purposes

- **Diagnostic nerve block:** to identify the exact source of pain

- **Nerve conduction:** to find nerve damage

- **Thermographic imaging:** to assess circulation

- **Discography:** to determine whether pain is originating from discs

- **Functional anesthestic discography (FAD):** to confirm the presence of injured discs

- **Magnetic resonance imaging (MRI):** to scan internal structures

- **Computerized axial tomography (CAT):** to show a detailed view of internal organs

- **Evoked potential:** to locate affected muscles or nerves

- **Psychological testing:** to assess emotional factors

- **X-rays:** to look for problems in bones and joints

[from Cleveland Clinic Pain Management Department]

APPENDIX I: RESOURCES

In addition to local and regional pain clinics, organizations and self-help groups, there are agencies at the national level that directly or indirectly provide services for people with chronic pain. Below is the contact information for 28 of those agencies.

Cleveland Clinic Dept. of Pain Management
10524 Euclid Avenue
Cleveland, OH 44195
1.800.223.2273
www.clevelandclinic.org/painmanagement

American Academy of Pain Management
13947 Mono Way #A
Sonora, CA 95370
1.209.533.9744
www.aapainmanage.org

American Academy of Medical Acupuncture (AAMA)
1970 E. Grand Avenue, Suite 330
El Segundo, California 90245
1.310.364.0193
www.medicalacupuncture.org

American Academy of Orthopaedic Surgeons
6300 North River Road
Rosemont, Illinois 60018-4262
1.847.823.7186
www.aaos.org

American Academy of Pain Medicine
4700 W. Lake Avenue
Glenview, IL 60025
1.847.375.4731
www.painmed.org

American Cancer Society
1599 Clifton Road, NE
Atlanta, GA 30329
1.800.227.2345
www.cancer.org

American Chiropractic Association
1701 Clarendon Boulevard
Arlington, VA 22209
1.703.276.8800
www.amerchiro.org

American Chronic Pain Association (ACPA)
PO Box 850
Rocklin, CA 95677-0850
1.800.533-3231
www.theacpa.org

American Headache Society Committee for Headache Education (ACHE)
19 Mantua Road
Mt. Royal, NJ 08061
1.856.423.0043
www.achenet.org

American Pain Foundation
201 North Charles Street, Suite 710
Baltimore, MD 21201-4111
1.888.615.7246 (PAIN)
www.painfoundation.org

American Pain Society
4700 W. Lake Avenue
Glenview, IL 60025
1.847.375.4715
www.ampainsoc.org

American Society of Regional Anesthesia and Pain Medicine (ASRA)
520 N. Northwest Highway
Park Ridge, IL 60068-2573
1.847.825.7246
www.asra.com

Arthritis Foundation
PO Box 7669
Atlanta, GA 30357
1.800.283.7800
www.arthritis.org

Fibromyalgia Network
PO Box 31750
Tucson, AZ 85751-1750
1.800.853.2929
www.fmnetnews.com

IBS Self Help & Support Group
24 Dixwell Avenue #118
New Haven, CT 06511
1.203.404.0660
www.ibsgroup.org

International Pelvic Pain Society
Two Woodfield Lake
1100 E. Woodfield Road, Suite 520
Schaumburg, IL 60173
Tel: 847-517-8712
www.pelvicpain.org

Mayday Fund
c/o SPG
127 West 26th St., Suite #800
New York, NY 10011
1.212.366.6970
www.maydayfund.org

NCCAM Clearinghouse
P. O. Box 7923
Gaithersburg, MD 20898
1.888.644.6226
www.nccam.nih.gov

**National Chronic Pain
Outreach Association (NCPOA)**
PO Box 274
Millboro, VA 24460
1.540.862.9437
www.chronicpain.org

**National Institute of Dental
and Craniofacial Research (NIDCR)**
National Institutes of Health
31 Center Drive, Room 5B-55
Bethesda, MD 20892
1.301.496.4261
www.nidcr.nih.gov

National Fibromyalgia Association
2121 S. Towne Centre Place, Suite 300
Anaheim, CA 92806
1.714.921.0150
www.fmaware.org

**National Foundation for
the Treatment of Pain**
1714 White Oak Drive
Houston, TX 77009
1.713.862.9332
www.paincare.org

National Headache Foundation
820 N. Orleans, Suite #217
Chicago, IL 60610-3132
1.888.643.5552
www.headaches.org

National Osteoporosis Foundation
1150 17th Street, NW, Suite #850
Washington, D.C. 20036
1.202.223.2226
www.nof.org

The Neuropathy Association
60 East 42nd Street, Suite #942
New York, NY 10165
1.212.692.0662
www.neuropathy.org

TMJ Association
PO Box 26770
Milwaukee, WI 53226-0770
1.262.432.0350
www.tmj.org

The Facial Pain Association
925 NW 56th Terrace, Suite C
Gainesville, FL 32605-6402
1.800.923.3608
www.fpa-support.org

World Institute of Pain (WIP)
145 Kimel Park Drive, Suite #310
Winston-Salem, NC 27103-6984
1.877.724.6360
www.worldinstituteofpain.org

APPENDIX II: GLOSSARY

acetaminophen — the basic ingredient found in Tylenol and equivalent drugs

analgesic — a class of drugs that includes most painkillers

anesthesia — medication that causes partial or complete loss of sensation, and sometimes loss of consciousness

anesthetic — a medicine that temporarily blocks pain

anticonvulsant — a drug used to prevent seizures that also can treat pain

antidepressant — any type of medicine used to treat depression

autonomic nervous system — the part of the nervous system that regulates involuntary body functions (such as the heart, circulation, and body temperature)

bioelectric treatment — a procedure in which a precise dose of bioelectric current is administered through electrodes placed on the skin to cause a biological change and interrupt pain signals

biomarker — a characteristic that is measured and evaluated as an indicator of normal or disease process

capsaicin — a chemical found in chili peppers that is the primary ingredient in many pain-relieving creams

central nervous system — the part of the nervous system made up of the brain and spinal cord

chronic pelvic pain syndrome — dull, sharp, steady, or intermittent pain that persists or recurs in the pelvic region over a period of weeks or months

cognitive behavioral therapy — a method of therapy that attempts to correct ingrained patterns of negative behaviors and thoughts

corticosteroid (steroid) — medication used to treat inflammation

cortisol — a hormone produced by the adrenal glands that decreases inflammation

COX-2 inhibitor — a nonsteroidal anti-inflammatory drug (NSAID) that is used to treat pain and reduce inflammation

discography — a procedure to determine whether an abnormal disc is causing pain

drug pump — a device placed under the skin to deliver extremely small doses of medication, usually to the space around the spinal cord that contains fluid

endorphins — naturally occurring molecules that attach to receptors in the brain and spinal cord to stop pain messages

epidural — a procedure used to provide anesthesia during childbirth and some types of surgery

evoked potential — a diagnostic test used to record the speed of nerve signal transmission to the brain

facet joint — a joint between two adjacent vertebrae

ibuprofen — an analgesic and NSAID that is sold over-the-counter and by prescription

immune system — the system responsible for protecting the body from disease

inflammation — the response of body tissues to injury or irritation

intractable pain — pain that does not respond to treatment

intrathecal — fluid-containing space around the spinal cord

limbic — the part of the brain that produces emotions

local anesthetic — a medication that blocks electrical signals and eliminates pain in a specific part of the body

myofascial pain — pain in the muscles and adjacent fibrous tissues

narcotics (opioids) — drugs that relieve pain by preventing transmission of pain messages to the brain

nerve block — the use of drugs, chemical agents, or a surgical procedure to interrupt the transmission of pain messages

neuralgia — pain that extends along nerve pathways

neurolytic — a substance or procedure that destroys nerve tissue

neuropathic pain — pain caused by injury to or inflammation of the nerves

neurostimulation — electrical pulses delivered by an implanted device to stimulate the spinal cord

neurotransmitters — substances in the brain that carry signals between nerve cells

nociceptive (somatic) pain — pain caused by tissue damage in which chemicals are released and perceived by the brain as pain

nociceptor — a specialized nerve ending that senses unpleasant sensations

non-neuropathic pain — pain that does not involve nerve damage

nonsteroidal anti-inflammatory drug (NSAID) — a drug used to reduce inflammation (aspirin and ibuprofen are examples)

opioids (narcotics) — drugs that relieve pain by preventing transmission of pain messages to the brain

pain patch — a covering containing medication that is applied to the skin to relieve pain

pain receptor — a specialized nerve ending that identifies painful sensations and transmits them to a nerve

palliative care — treatment to relieve the pain, symptoms, and stress of serious illness, regardless of the diagnosis or prognosis

patient controlled analgesia (PCA) — a system in which a person pushes a button and a machine delivers a dose of pain medicine into his or her bloodstream

peripheral nerve stimulation — a type of pain relief that uses electrical signals from an implanted device to stimulate nerves outside of the spine

peripheral nervous system — the part of the nervous system that lies outside the brain and spinal cord

phantom pain — pain following amputation that feels as if it comes from the missing limb

placebo — a harmless, inactive substance that has no direct effect on the cause of pain

sciatica — a painful condition caused by pressure on the sciatic nerve that causes pain in the buttocks, thighs, legs, ankles, and feet

serotonin — a chemical in the brain that helps to regulate mood

somatic (nociceptive) pain — pain caused by tissue damage in which chemicals are released and perceived by the brain as pain

spinal cord stimulation — electrical stimulation of nervous tissues in a specific portion of the spinal cord known as the dorsal column

SSRIs (selective serotonin reuptake inhibitors) — medications used to relieve depression that may also indirectly relieve pain

stenosis — narrowing of the canal surrounding the spinal cord

steroid — medication used to treat inflammation

subcutaneous — beneath the skin

sympathetic nervous system — one of two divisions of the autonomic nervous system that controls many of the involuntary activities of the glands, organs, and other parts of the body

syndrome — a group of symptoms that indicate a particular disorder

thalamus — the part of the brain that relays impulses from the nerves and enables people to feel pain

thermography — a measurement of heat produced by different parts of the body

topical drugs — medications that are applied to the skin

transdermal — a substance that enters the body through the skin

transcription therapy — treating conditions, including chronic pain, by introducing engineered genes into a patient's cells

tricyclic antidepressants — a group of drugs used to relieve symptoms of depression that may also relieve pain

trigger point — a specific spot that is painful to touch or pressure

X-STOP — a minimally-invasive procedure in which an implant is used to maintain the space between the spinous processes to prevent pressure on the nerves while standing